IT'S
Different
FOR
Men

IT'S
Different
FOR
Men

THE **MEN'S WEIGHT-LOSS** STRATEGY FOR **HEALTH,** **WEALTH,** AND **SEXUAL VITALITY**

HARVEY BROOKER

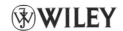

WILEY

John Wiley & Sons Canada, Ltd.

Library and Archives Canada Cataloguing in Publication Data

Brooker, Harvey
    It's different for men : the men's weight-loss strategy for health, wealth, and sexual vitality/Harvey Brooker.

Includes index.
ISBN 978-0-470-15391-8

    1. Weight loss. 2. Men—Nutrition. 3. Men—Health and hygiene.
I. Title.

RM222.2.B784 2008   613.2′5081   C2008-900611-9

Production Credits
Cover and interior text design: Jason Vandenberg
Typesetting: Thomson Digital
Printer: Friesens

John Wiley & Sons Canada, Ltd.
6045 Freemont Blvd.
Mississauga, Ontario
L5R 4J3

Printed in Canada

1 2 3 4 5 FP 12 11 10 09 08

Barb, my sister; Ida, my mom; and Dave, my dad. . . .
I think about you every day.

"Only those who can see the invisible can achieve the impossible."

CONTENTS

ACKNOWLEDGMENTS

It's been said that "when the students are ready the teacher will arrive," but in my career of helping men to change their course of life by changing how they think about food, I've learned that the real truth has been "when the teacher is ready, the students will arrive."

Every time another man asks me to help him learn to change, I realize what a gift I have been given. Through my words and example, and through my client's determination and tenacity, miracles take place. Hopelessness turns into hope, and new lives are carved from those that often seemed headed for an uncertain and perhaps diseased-filled future.

The men who are part of my world today can take comfort in the fact that this practitioner, this learner, their mentor and coach, has benefited from the lessons of all those who came before them.

In 1971, my wife Helen and I started the Toronto branch of a Boston-based franchise, the Diet Workshop. There were about 99 women for every man attending. Within the first year, a man called Bob, who was one of our original male clients, lost about 100 pounds.

Maybe 10 years later, Bob called me from the intensive care ward of the Branson Hospital here in Toronto. He had gained all his weight back and then some, and he was pleading with me to help him. He had type 2 diabetes and had already had his leg removed. He was scared. To this day, I can still hear the tremor in his voice.

I knew that by that stage, there was nothing that anyone could have done for Bob. He died just a few days after our conversation. That unspeakable tragedy shook me and changed me forever.

I had to ask myself, "What about all the other Bobs?" Who was going to help them? I've had Bob's words—"Harvey, please can you help me?"—in my ears ever since.

In November 1985, I began working exclusively with men. There was little a man could do in those days; after all, it was thought, a fat person was a fat person, and the differences in gender really didn't matter. That thinking was wrong then, and it is wrong now. There is a difference when it comes to losing our weight and changing our lives.

This book is dedicated to my clients, to Bob, and to all the other guys who just want someone to show them a lasting way to a healthier and slimmer life.

I've been given a talent, the ability to speak about my calling with a passion. I do that every Sunday morning at 10 a.m. None of this would have been possible without the support and strength of my good friend Terry Howes, who after losing 60 pounds with me about 20 years ago, has been on a mission to make certain that I keep the group going no matter what.

In 1994 Terry placed ads in the local newspapers to try to bring more men to the all-men's group. He paid for these ads out his own pocket. Thanks, Terry, for your belief in me.

My teachers have been many. My buddy Raymond Aaron came to me to learn how to live a healthier life in 1999. After losing 50 pounds himself, he sold me on continuing my learning by joining his wonderful program, The Monthly Mentor. Thanks, Raymond; you've shown me that everything is possible.

At this point in my career, I have worked with more than a thousand men, some who "got it" right away and some who were slower to see the way to a better life. I have learned from each and every one of them.

I believe I will be learning and growing to the last day of my life, and I will keep searching for answers to help men see that they don't have to settle for their current state of health and obesity.

This book is dedicated to all men. There is some in-your-face attitude in these pages that you may feel is unreasonable at first, but I hope that in time, you will get the point. These pages will help you to change the course of your life for the better. Always remember that the power to do this is in you, never give up or give in.

I would like to thank my friend Rick Gossage, who believed in this book and felt we could bring my philosophies to a bigger audience of men.

I would also like to thank Leah Marie Fairbank, who helped to organize my life's work so that it would fit concisely into these pages.

Special thanks to Patti Plant for her personal support of me and my program.

I want to recognize the Sunday crew who make my life so much easier by being there for me each and every week. Marlene Rumanak, our friend whose smiling face and pleasant character is comforting for all the men who come to us each week. Our volunteers—Ben Bijak, Charles O'Neil, Stephen Rath, Don Oates, Nick Ellis, Walter Dobko, Eric Cohen, Richard Burton, Oscar Orellana, Michael Kohnle, Peter Dunst, and Marty Roy, who said, "*Believe that you can and find out how along the way.*"

To my children, David, Evan, and Felicia, and their families, whose ongoing love and support continue to provide me with motivation to work to make other men's lives as happy as mine. I thank you every day.

And finally, I thank my life partner and my best friend, Helen, who always believed in me and gave me strength to keep moving in the direction of my dreams.

Harvey A. Brooker
Toronto, 2007

INTRODUCTION

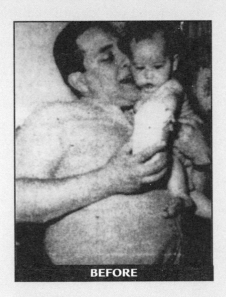

BEFORE

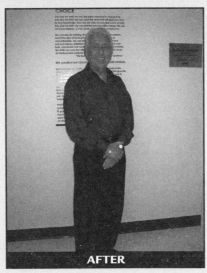

AFTER

COULD THIS BE YOU?

- Are you the guy standing at the back of all your family photos, so that only your neck and head will be in the picture? Or are you the guy who always volunteers to take the picture so that you can completely avoid being in it?
- Do you notice your reflection in the store window and think, "That can't be me"?

- Do you think that you're not *that* fat, but for some time you've been gaining a bit more weight each year?
- Have you been putting on weight as a result of stress related to a domestic break-up? A loss in your family? A business setback?
- Is frustration over the behavior of a particular child causing you to make trips to the refrigerator?
- Are you now at the stage where you finish all the food that is left by everyone else at every meal?
- Have you noticed that you have less and less energy?
- Do you have older clothes that you really like, and you just can't get into them anymore?
- Have you been gaining weight every year and you keep thinking someday you'll do something about it?
- Have you run into an old school chum on the street and he simply didn't recognize you?
- Are you the guy who used to be a jock and now all you can do is watch sports?
- Do you find that you can't fit into a booth in a restaurant and need to find a chair?
- Are you the guy who used to walk the golf course and can't anymore?
- Do you find yourself using the second stair to mount your foot so you can bend down to tie up your own shoelaces? Have you started to favor Velcro shoes?
- Does your neck bleed over your collar?
- Have you noticed that you are wearing your belt farther and farther below your 'real' waist?
- When you're at a public event, do you have to sit the entire time with your arms crossed because you don't want to spill your neighbor's drink?
- When you walk down the aisle of the plane, do you sense people thinking, "Thank god he's not sitting next to me"?

- Are you the guy that goes to the beach and parks himself in a chair?
- Have you hit the stage where you won't wear sweaters because you don't want to show your boobs?
- After dieting, do you keep your large clothes because you know in your heart that you'll need them again?
- At one time, did women find you attractive and now they don't look back anymore?
- Do you sit in the end seat at a baseball game or movie theatre? Or, worse yet, you just can't fit in those seats, so you don't go to plays or movies anymore?
- Are you the guy that can't sit in the airplane without a seat belt extension? And when the snacks come, the tray from the seat in front of you won't go flat because it hits your stomach?
- Do you ask your company to pay for first class air tickets, because those are the only seats that you can fit into?
- Do you get your partner to attend the PTA meeting because your child told you that he was embarrassed about how you looked?
- Are you concerned that you won't last until your daughter's wedding? Are you worried about what others will think when you're escorting her down the aisle?
- Are you now rolling out of bed because you can't sit up?
- Are you the guy that has found himself dozing at a stoplight because of sleep apnea?
- Are you the guy that forces his wife to live with a Continuous Positive Airway Pressure (CPAP) machine?
- Do you wake up in the middle of the night with the burning sensation of heartburn or night sweats?
- Are you the guy who inevitably regurgitates his meal when he lies down?
- When people see you in the front of the elevator, do they wait for the next one?
- Do your bowel movements hurt?

- Have you been having excruciating pain in your big toe due to gout?
- Do you find that you're chronically short of breath?
- Do you hear the same thing every time you go to the doctor: "If you don't lose the weight, 10 years from now you'll be dead"?
- Are you worried that you're going to die early, because your father did?
- Are you the boy who called wolf by telling your friends that you were going to lose weight permanently and didn't?
- Are you too embarrassed to tell them whenever you try again?
- Have you spent enough money on weight loss books without finding an answer for men?

I had. In fact, I'd spent a lot of my life going through a lot of these awkward situations and more! By my mid-twenties, I'd packed 215 pounds onto a five-foot-six-inch frame. I'll never let myself forget those times, because all of that embarrassment and humiliation has provided me with the motivation to eat properly for the rest of my life.

Like the majority of overweight men—and possibly like you—I did not start off fat. I was an active and skinny little kid, running around and playing hard, and never even thinking about food.

According to my Aunt Gerty, who lived with our extended family, I was too skinny, and she determined to do something about it. Her understanding was that men were supposed to be big. While we were by no means rich, we always had a lot of food in the house, and she saw to it that I ate as much as possible. I discovered that I really liked the taste of food! It was only later I realized that we had a very fattening diet: brisket, cabbage rolls, knishes, and other delightful dishes—many of them cooked in schmaltz or rendered chicken fat.

When I suffered the trauma of my father's death, at the young age of 12, I remembered my time with my aunt. She had taught me that food was one four-letter word that represented another four-letter word: love. I used food to console myself. Unfortunately, as I got over the loss I continued to eat excessively because I'd learned to love it.

All this food made me fat. I can remember my embarrassment when I was taken to Eaton's Department Store. I was mortified to discover that I could not get new clothing in the children's section but had to be redirected to the "husky" department.

Yet the change did not come for many more years. My wife and I were at the theatre; we had gone to see the musical *Hair*. Very risqué, for those days! I remember vividly that my shirt was squeezing me so tightly it made me feel like I had to go to the bathroom. Unfortunately, I couldn't leave my seat because of the trim, virtually nude bodies running up and down the theatre aisles. And, as I turned to see the actors behind me, I popped all the buttons on my shirt. There I was in a public place with my stomach hanging out.

I pulled my sports jacket across to try and cover up the disaster. I felt humiliated and disgusted with myself. I could hardly watch the play as I worried about how I would make a graceful exit from the theatre after the lights came back on. The pain and embarrassment cut so deep that I was absolutely determined to change. I vowed then and there to take the weight off, and to do it permanently. I was 26 years old. If I'd continued eating the way I always had, I would probably have died within 20 years.

I lost the weight over a period of time with the Weight Watchers organization. Later, I worked for their company and others, but they were always focused on women's weight loss. My own remembered humiliation was so strong, I didn't care if I was the only man in the room; but that isn't the case with most men, and it doesn't need to be. Men need to learn what affects their physiology, their eating habits, and their weight. They need to know how to control their weight—on their own terms.

I taught my first class to men in 1985, and I have never looked back. Since then, I've conducted more than 32,000 half-hour one-on-one coaching sessions with men and conducted over 1,100 men-only support groups.

Over these 30-plus years, I've learned that it really is "Different for Men." I've learned things about weight that no one's ever told you before. This isn't about tight abs, like you see on the front of a men's health magazine. It's not about a diet that works temporarily, only to make you gain more weight when it ends. This book is about your life and how you can eliminate the very dramatic risks associated with excess weight. In every page, I've tried to provide unvarnished thoughts that will help you sort through the crap that's out in the marketplace and understand how you can stop being a statistic in the rapidly increasing numbers of obese men in industrialized countries. You'll meet men in the pages of the book who have permanently changed their lives. And you can do it, too.

There is a reason why you're overweight, and there is a reason why the other weight loss programs won't work for you. Losing weight is an equal combination of choosing the right food and finding the motivation to make a permanent change in your lifestyle. I believe strongly that if you're motivated enough to read this book, then you're motivated and capable enough to change your life! You just need to see a path through the forest of food temptations that will never leave you hungry. It's a path that I walk every day, and so will you.

PART 1

IT'S DIFFERENT FOR MEN

IF I EAT THE SAME WAY, WHY DO I KEEP GAINING?

1

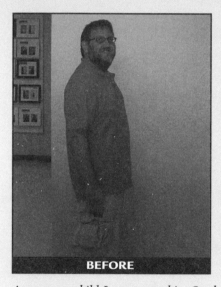

BEFORE

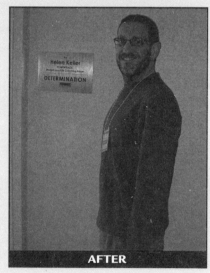

AFTER

As a young child I was very thin. So thin, in fact, that my parents gave me appetite stimulation medication. I suppose the medicine worked really, really well! From around the age of eight, I began to have a weight problem. I went from a chubby kid, to a heavy teen, to an overweight young adult, and was embarrassed at what I had become by the time I heard about Harvey Brooker's men's weight loss program. For many years, I had avoided my "annual" medical check-up because I did not want to be told that I needed to lose some weight. I knew that I should lose weight. I knew that my eating was out of control. Trying to lose weight was my life's theme until I was in my mid-thirties. Then I gave up. I decided that

I should "accept myself for who I am." Being overweight had become who I was. Why fight it? I decided to buy larger clothes and try to "enjoy" life.

By the time I turned 40, I was well past 200 pounds. I was not enjoying life. In fact, there was a small voice in my head that kept telling me that I was killing myself. By the summer of 2006, I took the proverbial look at myself in the mirror and decided that if I wanted to see my children grow up I needed to do something. That's when I heard about Harvey Brooker's program. I went to a meeting and knew right away that this was the program for me. The program made sense. I spent 38 years of my life proving that I could not control my eating. "Treating myself" with just a bit of ice cream always led to overindulgence. Chicken wings, fries, and pizza had brought me to where I was. Dieting never worked for me; eventually the diet ended.

The Harvey Brooker program was different. It was not a diet. It was a program that, once mastered, could continue throughout my life. It has now been 15 months since I started the program and I am proud to say that I am in total control of my weight. How has it changed my life? I feel like I am going to live for a very long time. I feel like I am a positive role model to my children.

Jordan Hoffman

You're reading this book because, on some level, you realize you weigh more than you should. If you're honest, your weight is probably increasing every year.

In fact, you are probably gaining more and more weight in spite of the fact that you're eating the same amount of food as 20 or 30 years ago. Here's the wake-up call: unless you change your eating behavior, you will continue to gain more rapidly every year.

The ground was probably laid back when you were that young man with boundless energy. In those days you got into the habit of having greasy lunches on the run. You also drank quite a lot of soft drinks and beer. You never thought about what you ate or how much you ate, because it didn't seem to matter. You were still growing, and you were still exercising frequently. For a while it seemed like you couldn't gain weight, and if you did, it would be gone again after summer break. Unfortunately, this is where your bad eating habits were becoming really engrained, never again to be questioned.

If you went to university or college, it was easy and very convenient for you to be engaged in team sports. You may have lived on campus, the facilities were right there, and your roommates or friends were also participating. You were gaining some weight, but doesn't everyone "fill out" at this stage? What you didn't realize was that even with regular exercise, your body couldn't handle the overload of sugars, carbs, huge portions, and late eating that were becoming your life. So the weight crept up.

When you started working, all of a sudden you spent most days sitting down; 175 pounds gradually became 190 pounds. You had a little less energy, but you still played pick-up basketball once or twice a week or maybe the odd game of tennis on the weekend.

At some point, your meals became more regular, although you didn't have time for breakfast before going to work—you wanted to stay as long as you could in bed with your partner. You made up for breakfast with a mid-morning muffin and coffee with cream. Your weight was now creeping up to 200 pounds.

Remember that promise that you had made to yourself that your weight would never go over 200? That you would never buy size 38 pants? Oh, well, you said to yourself—"When I get more established at my job, I'll have time to go to the gym and sweat it off." In the meantime, you also noticed that your appetite had increased and that even when you did allow time for a proper breakfast, you still had that muffin mid-morning. Work could be frustrating, but you were finding relaxation and relief with a few drinks and then a steak frites dinner with a bottle of wine.

Chances are that as you slid down this track, you decided to fight back, but like most other men, you never thought about changing what you ate. Instead, you made a concerted effort to go to the gym. You were only able to sweat off five pounds.

By the age of 40, you're losing the battle. You're now 30 or 40 or 100 or more pounds overweight, and the weight gain has become a runaway train.

If your 20-year-old self could see you right now, would he recognize you? If he could talk to you at this moment, he'd probably say, "How could you have let this happen to me? You used to be able to leap over walls with unstoppable energy and now, in your early forties, you weigh in at 245 and you're exhausted. Worse yet, you have high blood pressure and your cholesterol is way up!"

WHERE ARE YOU HEADED?

Get yourself a pencil and paper, and record your weight from 20 years ago. Then write down what it was 10 years ago, five years ago and finally write down what you weigh today. Now make a graph with your age in years along the bottom and your weight up the side. Mark in your numbers with X's and project the curve of the line out five years, and then 10 years, and take a look at what's ahead.

What you're going through is, unfortunately, all too normal. Hundreds, perhaps thousands, of men have come to me with the same story: 20 years ago they had a few extra pounds, and today they are 60 or 100 or 200 pounds overweight.

The big question is *why?*

You gain weight because of your previous weight gain.

As you grow older, your weight gain generally comes from adding fat to your body. Fat tissues do not use as much energy as muscle tissues, so you use fewer and fewer calories over time.

If the majority of your weight is made up of fat, rather than muscle, and you continue to take in the same amount of calories, you're taking in more than your body needs, and you gain weight. You have to combine diet and exercise in order to lose weight effectively; exercise on its own will not do the trick.

The longer you carry around excess weight, and the older you get, the more immobile you become, the more stress you place on your weight-bearing joints, and the more you will gain—even if you eat the same amount as before. This is not just a weight problem, but a structural and physics problem.

Here is the calculation to use if you're interested in where you are headed:

> Take the weight gain that you've had in the past five years and multiply it by 1.5. For example, let's say today you weigh 250 pounds, and five years ago you weighed 230 (and of course you promised yourself you would never weigh over 230). You gained 20 pounds. If you don't take action, in five years your weight gain will be 1.5 times that number—another 30 pounds. You will be 280 pounds. Five years after that? 325.

Along with the extra weight gain comes an exponential increase in all the associated diseases and chronic symptoms—high blood pressure, high cholesterol, sleep apnea, type 2 diabetes, lack of sex drive. And it's not only physical: your work life will suffer too, because of decreased energy and diminished self-esteem.

Today, you may not find yourself as far along this dangerous path as I have described. Maybe you're only 25 pounds over your ideal weight, and you'd like to get your younger, more athletic body back. You're not really that concerned about obesity.

I've seen the pattern repeated often enough to know that if you continue your eating habits without a ONE80-degree change in your behavior, there will come a point in your life when the weight gain curve (if you were graphing it) will become exponential. It will shoot straight towards the top of the page.

If someone made you wear a 25-pound wetsuit and you had to walk around with it all day, you'd tell them to get lost. You'd think that such an effort would be stupid and exhausting. Yet by gaining 15 or 25 pounds, that's exactly what you're asking your body to do. You will become more and more sedentary, not just from poor food choices and digestive exhaustion, but also from the growing effort it takes to move around.

Your muscles and joints have to move that extra weight wherever you go, every waking moment, causing your knee and hip joints to wear out. Inevitably, you will slow down, and of course, because you're eating the same amount of the same kind of food, you'll find it that much easier to gain the next 10 pounds, and it will happen even more quickly. This momentum will soon start to feed on itself. This is what I call the exponential weight gain syndrome.

Here's an imaginary situation: You're 20 years old and a college or university student. You weigh 185 pounds on a five-foot-eleven frame. Your energy is boundless. You walk around campus all day and have enough energy for a pick-up football game when classes end. If there's a party that night you go dancing. Everything seems effortless. When you finally crash into bed at midnight (okay, 3:00 a.m.) you fall asleep instantly, and only wake up when the alarm is ringing for the third time.

Bring your thoughts forward to how you feel today. Think about how much effort it takes to do the simplest things. You're out of energy from walking up the stairs. You feel ancient when you get in and out of the car. You don't sleep well. Would that young guy understand or recognize the overweight gentleman who's sitting here reading this book right now?

At what moment did it get away from you, and why? How do you change the direction? You might blame it on your metabolism—"It's slower than it used to be." Or is it the fault of family genetic traits? "My Uncle Louis was fat!"

Right now, whether your weight is 20 pounds over your ideal or 120 pounds over, a permanent solution is necessary.

Why don't you take another look at that graph that I asked you to create? Think for a minute about how high that line could rise, and how quickly that could happen. Do you want to take that chance?

Now imagine what you'd like to be doing with your life in five years. What are your work goals? How would you like to be spending time? With your family? With your friends? Traveling?

Given your health at this moment, and the trajectory that you can see on the graph you've just drawn, what are your chances of being able to do those things?

If you continue on this route, how do you think your employer and your family and friends will relate to you? Will you still be able to participate at the same level in these different roles? If the answer is "I won't," then it's time you changed your life ONE80 degrees. If the answer is "I might not even be alive in five years if I continue on this route," then change is the only choice a reasonable man would make.

You can do what I did—and what I've helped thousands of men to do. I can show you how to raise your self-esteem without pills and without hunger by giving you the confidence to try, by giving you a workable plan to follow, and by having you eat the right quantities of ordinary, readily available, satisfying foods. The men that you see throughout this book had all failed before and yet were able to permanently turn their lives around. I'm sure that when you've finished reading this book, you will know in your heart that you can join my group of successes.

Your first goal should be to stop the trend toward obesity and an early death. Your next goal is to reverse it. You can do this with three easy components: 1) a sensible, sustainable eating plan; 2) exercise; and 3) support.

You can't do this alone. If you could, you would have done it by now. There's no shame in admitting that you need help along the way. But you also can't keep going the way you have been. Something's gotta give.

It's time to move forward on a different path, a path that leads to permanent weight loss and the best health of your life. The results will be good news for your body, your career, your sex life—and your self-esteem.

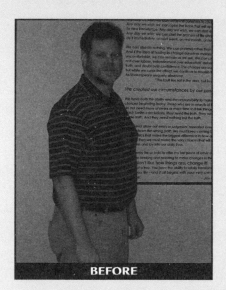

BEFORE

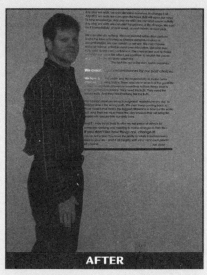

AFTER

Clearly, I wasn't as smart as I thought I was. Although I've been overweight all of my adult life, I've always kidded myself that I was only a quick fad diet away from losing the extra pounds. I had been marginally successful with all of them at one point in my life or another: 25 pounds under the Eat-Nothing-but-Cheese-Eggs-and-Bacon diet; 20 pounds under the Sure-You-Can-Have-Chocolate-Cake-on-This-Diet-but-Just-TRY-to-Stop-at-One-Piece diet; 30 pounds under the No-Breakfast-No-Lunch-Stuff-Yourself-Silly-at-Night diet; and so on, each time gaining back more than I had lost.

In recent years I was averaging a five- to seven-pound weight gain every year, looking worse and worse, and feeling like hell. I needed a new pair of jeans each spring, and I would stretch my shirts out of shape, hoping I'd be able to fit into them for a few more months before sheepishly buying new ones at yet another size larger. Nevertheless, I would still lie to myself again and again that I could easily change things by plugging into the next fad for a few weeks.

In September 2006, my wife, Anna, and I were blessed with the birth of two wonderful children, Polly and Angus. I vowed then that I would use the winter to get back into shape.

On the contrary, I found that the stress and sleeplessness associated with infant twins was turning me towards—and not away from—the fatty, sugary junk that I had sworn off. By the time they were eight months old, I had gained 12 pounds. Simple math was telling me that by the time they got to high school, their father would be over 300 pounds.

In early May, I woke up from a dream that I have not forgotten and will try not to ever forget: In the dream, Polly and Angus are about seven or eight and they are called into the school principal's office. The principal tells them that they can go home from school early today because their father's heart has exploded. "He cared more about french fries and pizza and cake and ice cream than he cared about you and so he is leaving you." That week I joined Harvey Brooker's weight loss group for men.

At my first meeting, I met several fellows who had lost 50-100 pounds and more and had kept it off! I was introduced to a guy who looked for all the world to me like a slim fellow, completely out of place at a weight-loss meeting. He'd lost 80 pounds two years earlier and yet was still attending. He called himself a "one-percenter," explaining that only one percent of people who lose significant weight manage to keep it off for more than a year. Boy, did that ever sound familiar. Turned out Harvey's group had lots of one-percenters!

Harvey came out to speak and, shockingly, offered no easy solutions. He spoke honestly and told me things that deep down I always knew but denied to myself:

- *That I'm not going to lose weight by pretending that I can continue to eat the food that made me fat;*
- *That there are situations that I just can't handle in terms of eating and I must control them or avoid them altogether; and*
- *That the changes I make now I must make for the rest of my life because I can never stop at just one cookie, or just one chicken wing, or just one slice of pizza.*

I hit my goal weight within four months and have surpassed it by an additional 15 pounds. I have discovered the true shape of my body: I had always assumed I was a big-boned guy who was fat; in fact, I am a small-framed guy who was really fat! And while of course I am proud of how I look and thrilled with the way my new clothes hang on me, I am most grateful to Harvey for helping me discover all of the life and energy I have within me. I can now state confidently that, as they grow up, my children need not worry about their father's health or whether he'll have the energy to get off the couch to play with them, or attend their games or be with them at the important times of their lives. I can't see how I could ever thank Harvey enough for that gift.

Bruce MacDonald

There are many issues that are entirely particular to our own sex that contribute to men being overweight. This chapter will examine the realities of our everyday existence and the unique factors that cause us to gain weight. Understanding how you got to where you are now will make it possible for you to see exactly where you need to go.

MEN GAIN WEIGHT AROUND THE ABDOMEN

When men put on weight, it's almost inevitably around the abdomen. You've seen the look: guys with their belts cinched up to hold everything in place. If you measure your waist below this protrusion, the measurement doesn't change much over time; you can fool yourself into believing you aren't gaining weight.

Why don't you take a test? Put a measuring tape around your body so that it is parallel to the floor and goes across your belly button. This is your actual waist circumference, regardless of the size of the last pair of pants you bought.

Some people call it a beer belly and some a spare tire, but it amounts to the same thing. And it's not only unattractive; it's dangerous. Excess fat around the waist means excess fat around your organs, and that creates very real health hazards, including heart disease, type 2 diabetes, and poor sexual function.

MEN ARE CONDITIONED TO WANT CERTAIN FOODS

What is "men's food"? Picture in your head a meal "fit for a king." Be honest: did a salmon fillet with rice just pop to mind, or a huge mountain of steak? Men eat way too much red meat and protein in general. Because of this, most menus describe the protein part of the course—everything else is an afterthought. Conditioned attitudes toward food like this help to explain the success of major restaurant chains that offer heaping plates with little nutrition. Left unchallenged, this kind of eating continues to cause men significant health problems in later life.

MEN ARE ENCOURAGED TO EAT AND DRINK TOO MUCH

Men are expected to eat much more than woman and are served proportionately way too much, especially too much protein. We learn to eat a lot when we are young; we're told it's "manly" and that we need to eat as much as we can because we're growing. (In my case, it didn't matter whether I was hungry or not: I was coached to eat. When I cleaned a plate and I was stuffed like a Thanksgiving turkey, I got a 25-cent reward from my Aunt Gerty.) Then it simply becomes a habit. And others get onboard as well. Our friends and partners and parents continue to offer us the largest plate, and we accept. Because we eat it, they offer it again the next time, and the trend continues.

The same is true of drinking. Our buddies inevitably offer the extra scotch, beer, or glass of wine. More often than not, we accept the extra drink or two (or six), because, unlike most women, men are woefully naïve about the number of empty calories that they consume through alcohol.

MEN AREN'T TAUGHT TO THINK ABOUT THEIR WEIGHT

Until a man's weight affects his health, sex life, or job, he is probably not going to pay any attention to what's happening. When was the last time you heard some guys sitting around together discussing that latest diet, or how they were going to fit into a particular suit? "Honey, do I look all right in this?" Big guys are big guys, right? They're lucky because they can eat and drink more, right? Unfortunately, this means weight gain progresses a lot farther before we start trying to do something about it, and we've got a lot farther to travel to get back to our ideal body type.

SOCIETY SEEMS TO BE FORGIVING OF OVERWEIGHT MEN

We all know that society pressures women to be thin. In business, politics, or on a date—women's bodies are regularly scrutinized. What happens for men is different. On the surface, men can carry around an extra thirty pounds and still find a mate, still own the company, still be president of the United States. This allows men to convince themselves that nothing is wrong, and that nothing needs to change.

However, on the deeper level, these men are spiraling toward ever more weight, ever decreasing energy, chronic disease, and early death. More than that, though we aren't *meant* to be worried about our weight, though we are *told* that society will grant power and love to an overweight man, the truth is very different. Overweight men are often passed over for promotion, often have more difficulty finding and keeping a life partner, and though they may not say it out loud, they almost always lack the confidence to get out there and do what they really want with their lives.

MEN'S MEDIA RARELY EXPOSES MEN TO FOOD, HEALTH, AND DIETARY ISSUES

Think about some popular magazines. Eliminate those magazines that are aimed at body builders and chronic gym buffs, and think about general interest men's magazines. Would *Outdoor Life* suggest a program to lose 10 pounds in two weeks? Imagine *Men's Journal* suggesting a weight loss program to get ready for the swimming season. Think about *Esquire* suggesting weight loss as a means of attracting that "right" woman. Imagine *Golf Digest* talking about a diet that would get you thin enough to walk around the golf course instead of riding in a cart!

The same is true about books. You can find out how to get washboard abs (dedicate your life to fitness), but every other aspect of health and fitness seems to be a subject only for women. How, then, are men to learn about their different physiology, about their different patterns of weight loss and gain—how are they to be successful in maintaining a healthy body?

MEN THINK THEY CAN WORK OFF CALORIES BY WORKING OUT

Exercise alone is not a replacement for proper eating habits. As you read through this book, you'll quickly realize that a couple of games a week of pick-up sport may be great for your social network, and your soul, but they don't make much difference to your waistline. Worse yet, these bonding endeavors are usually followed by pizza, or fries and beer, providing a calorie intake that more than cancels whatever benefit you achieved with your sporting activity.

MEN HAVE A SUPER BOWL (OR SUPER GUT) SUNDAY CULTURE

You can tell when these gatherings are about to occur. The cars arrive and everyone jumps out with a case of beer and some potato chips. Of course, it all goes together beautifully. Alcohol stimulates hunger, which stimulates eating the potato chips, which are covered in salt, which stimulates thirst, which stimulates drinking more beer. There are also nuts, nachos, salsa, cheezies, and buttery popcorn, all featuring lots of salt to keep you drinking. If the beer makes you sleepy, there's always Coke or Red Bull in the refrigerator. Men have big hands, and big hands make for big handfuls of this junk food.

Of course, you can't get full eating only these kinds of junk food, so along come the orders of wings and pizza, or wieners and burgers on the barbecue with white buns with lots of cheese (sometimes bacon), relish, ketchup, and mustard.

Men celebrate bad eating and they use bad eating to celebrate! It's a ritual that's been repeated in a similar way for generations, with one very important change in recent years: Full-time sports channels have changed what were occasional events (Super Bowl, World Series, World Cup) into a staggering number of weekly or even daily excuses to sit in front of the television. North American men can now spend *every* Saturday watching NCAA college football and *every* Sunday through the fall and early winter watching the NFL on their couch, and—you guessed it—eating junk food and drinking beer.

MEN THINK THEY CAN SWEAT IT OFF AT THE GYM

It used to work, right? A few weeks at the gym and all would be back to normal. Unfortunately, the gym alone is not your answer. Exercise is imperative for weight loss, but without proper nutrition you still run the risk of all the major chronic diseases associated with these eating habits (type 2 diabetes, heart disease, etc.). Further, you can't maintain your energy or fuel your body effectively. And men do not realize how much time they would need to spend in the gym to burn even a small portion of the calories that they are eating daily.

Exercise is great, and regular exercise will promote a feeling of well-being, and even help reduce your appetite, but exercise alone is not enough to get healthy and lose weight permanently.

MEN DON'T READ LABELS

Men are generally woefully ignorant of nutritional information. Try this: ask several of your male friends if they've ever read the details on the ingredients of any prepared food that they've bought. The chances are that they're going to look at you like you've lost your mind. Ask the same number of women, and there's a far better chance that they'll be able to tell you in general terms about the ingredients. A basic understanding of labels is crucial to weight management, so it's no wonder so many men continue to gain.

MEN THINK "DIETING" MEANS NOT EATING

A lack of nutritional knowledge leads to the common misperception that you can manage your weight by a balance of eating and not eating. The myth works like this: if you're going out for a big dinner later in the day, skip breakfast and lunch. If you ate a lot over the weekend, don't eat anything for the first couple of days of the next week.

What's the problem with this myth?

Going without food for even a short time tells your body that it's entering a famine, and all calories must be saved. The next meal you eat is immediately stored in case of further food shortages. It was a useful trait a few thousand years ago, but with food now constantly within arms' reach, it's dangerous. Though you may hate to think of it in these terms, you are actually "yo-yo dieting," causing short periods of weight loss followed by even more weight gain.

MEN WANT TO DO IT ALONE

Given our fixation on sports, I've never been able to figure out our belief that we don't need external support. All sports teams have specialty coaches.

Whether you play or not, you probably know that Tiger Woods is the best golfer in the world. Tiger Woods has a coach and the support of a team in order to be successful. You need a new set of skills to succeed at your weight loss—new knowledge, new dedication, new understanding—and you need support. The people closest to you are going to be involved in this, and that's a good thing for you. It's too easy to fall off the wagon, forget about making all this effort, and pick up another bag of takeout on the way home. It's too easy to blame it on someone else, or to privately suffer and publicly pretend everything is fine. You're happy to take golf lessons, because you know you won't improve without some expert help.

If you're overweight, I've always said that you have three choices: 1) Buy a farm and work it yourself; 2) keep gaining, or 3) follow the advice and use the support offered in this book. It's the same training I've been offering for more than 35 years, and it works.

MALE ANXIETY AND EATING

3

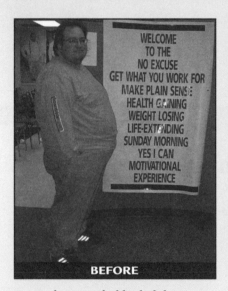

BEFORE

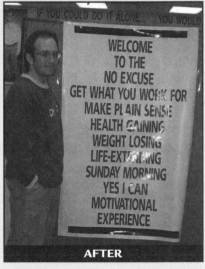

AFTER

I was always a chubby kid, but it was my introduction to teenage life and high school that saw me balloon to 420 pounds by my twenty-fourth birthday. My gift was being diagnosed with type 2 diabetes, and I got to start the roller coaster of trying to lose my weight. The medication worked for a bit, but I didn't really change my habits. The weight came back, slowly but surely. During this time, my dad got sick and passed away. He had always been the fit one in the house, so to see him falter was tough. You learn about your own mortality that way. Men in my dad's family die young. In their sixties. Was I going to make it there myself?

I sort of assigned myself to an early grave, without admitting it. It took a few more years of yo-yoing with my weight, adding the high blood pressure, fatigue, and high cholesterol to my growing accomplishments. Then one of the owners where I worked passed me the number for Harvey Brooker. After calling, I pushed off for a few weeks, until August 2004. I brought my brother to keep me company, and because I figured he needed the help too. I still had no idea what the program was; I assumed it was a one-time thing. But something clicked that day; Harvey really believed he could help us, and for the first time I think I really believed that I could actually get healthy. Never did I expect to lose as much as I did.

Losing 200 pounds was astonishing. I still cannot believe how much this has changed my life. I've got a great job that I believe I wouldn't have if I weighed 400 pounds, and I have a healthy outlook for myself and my brother (he lost 160 pounds), and a great future ahead.

Mike Kohnle

WHAT'S ON YOUR MIND?

Modern living has created a perfect storm for men: a dramatic decrease in physical activity, pre-packaged foods that contained tasty but nutrition-less ingredients—and a third factor. That factor is the way that many of us men were taught to behave as young boys.

Let's see if this socialization myth rings true for you. This myth is important to understand—and to debunk. Examining it will help you make sense of your own emotional state and make it easier to address the factors that will lead to permanent changes in your eating habits.

The myth is that *men are emotionally tough and have no feelings.* On some level, we all know that nothing could be farther from the truth. However, it is obvious that many men, perhaps most of us, do have difficulty expressing their emotions. The failure to express them to anyone often leaves them festering and unattended. The resulting pain can manifest itself in eating and drinking habits that lead to weight gain and potential obesity.

Most men grow up being told (usually by their fathers) to hide fear and hurt. The expression "Grow up and be a man" could just as easily be phrased "Learn to repress your feelings and emotions."

It starts early. If a young boy is injured, he's regularly told to "tough it out." Think back to when you fell off your bike or got kicked in the shins at a soccer game. Your dad's initial question was, "Are you all right?" The answer should have been obvious to him: "No, I'm not. Who's all right after being kicked in the shin?"

But you knew that this was not the expected or acceptable response. You had to summon up the Rambo that should be living in every little boy's soul. When you could catch your voice, you had to try and mumble "yes" even though you were sobbing. Then you were told, "Real men don't cry," or, "Just walk it off." If you were able to stem the tears quickly, and limp around until you worked your way through it, the other parents would applaud, and your teammates would high five you as you came off the field. Being tough earns you more respect.

This doesn't have to happen very often in early life for the idea to get through. The more you could hide misery, the more of a man you were. This continues into our adult lives.

This situation is exacerbated at work. If we became frustrated or annoyed there and broke into tears, without question, we would be shortening our careers. However, what happens if we get angry? Why, that's an entirely appropriate response for men!

I know successful men who get anxious at the thought of starting another week of work. They often turn to a big meal or cocktails on Sunday night just to get them through to the next day.

Many of us get so good at not showing our basic emotions that even when it's appropriate, or we really want to, we don't know how. So there we are at the birth of our son, our daughter's wedding, or the death of a parent and we don't know how to let go.

Long ago that outlet might have been for us to speak to one of the elders of the village. Later on, we might have spoken with a religious leader of some kind. I don't know about you, but I can't tell you who the elder of my village is, and I can't see myself going to speak with a politician. As for religious leaders, some individuals may call on them for help, but as organized religion becomes less and less the norm, we do this far less now than previous generations would have.

Some of us may talk to our friends about the issues that really concern us. It's my experience, however, that most men don't discuss the really sensitive parts of their lives with each other. Male bonding tends to be around sports, or drinking, or juvenile antics and pranks, but rarely about those things that really matter.

As a result, we're all at risk of going though a lifetime becoming progressively bottled up with anxiety. It doesn't matter whether the problems are real or imagined. We learn to keep everything balled up inside. All of us know that if we don't discuss the issues, we don't have the relief that might come from discovering that others have been feeling the same way. However, if you seem like the only one fighting a particular life battle then it can be a lonely and frightening position . . . and when you feel that anxiety, where do you look for the release?

A lot of men are full of rage. You can see it on the roads when you are driving. They want to get their lives back and yet they don't know how. If they are to exist in our modern world, they have to repress most of their human impulses. And what is a natural, human place to turn for release? Food. Yet men who turn to food for the answer find themselves in a very dangerous position.

I used to eat to defuse the stress of growing up in a dysfunctional family. There is no question in my mind that I turned to food to bring what I thought was pleasure into my life, but I quickly learned that it was a life that was out of control. The fact was that the solution had to come from dealing with the issues rather than eating to make myself feel better.

In my office, I do one-on-one counseling for men who are attempting to change. I probe the issues that my clients don't usually discuss: aging parents, sibling fears, unhappy marriages. The coaching always starts with a review of what the man is eating, but inevitably transfers into what is eating him. I keep a box of tissues in the office; you have no idea how many men break down when they start discussing their feelings about their obesity, and how they got there. Some of them have reached the stage where they can't clean themselves after going to the toilet because their arm isn't long enough for their altered body. I've had other men talk about how they were sexually abused as children and sought solace in food.

A man who loses control of his weight generally ends up loathing himself and feeling that he is losing his reason for living. If he's in this particular spiral, he's actually risking his life, and the worst part is that he's usually been so secretive about his feelings that he finds himself alone and without support. I've known and helped thousands of men like this. Men don't cry publicly, but I've had hundreds in tears in my office as they work their way through this unfortunate situation.

LOW SELF-ESTEEM

Even if you're only slightly overweight, you're beginning to drift from the ideal that you once were or that you could be. You can pretend on the outside that it doesn't matter, but it's a sign that you're beginning to lose control of your life. You know that others know this as well, and let's face it—that hurts.

How far you let it drift before you choose to act depends on how much reinforcement you're getting from other parts of your life. I had a client who described himself as "successfully fat." That meant that at least for a time in his overweight life he felt that he was getting away with overeating. His job was good, and his family was great. The problem with this thinking is that the more you let your weight get out of control, the more it affects all those other parts of your life that were propping up your self-image while you were letting your body deteriorate. Of course, my "successfully fat" client eventually came to me because he needed to do something to get his life back under control.

As you face any feelings of low self-worth, it's important to understand that you're not alone. If the statistics are telling the truth, then millions of men in North America are feeling the same way you do now.

So my message to you is simple. You are not alone if you have trouble expressing what you've been feeling about your life. You are not crazy because someone has prescribed you antidepressants. You're not demented because you have a lot of pent-up rage. You do have feelings and you're probably terribly frustrated, and if you're reading this chapter, possibly you've covered up a lot of these feelings by eating and drinking. And I'll bet the eating was focused on comfort food—sugars and fats in pre-packaged food that set you on a downward spiral.

As you will see in the next chapter, your self-esteem will affect your health, your work, and your sex life, so if you aren't feeling good about yourself, do something about it. Self-esteem can be restored as quickly as making an active decision to take control of your eating habits, and the good news is that getting control of your eating can help you master many of the other issues in your life.

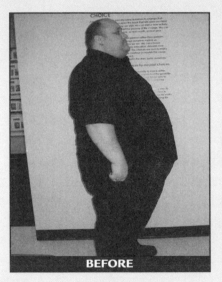 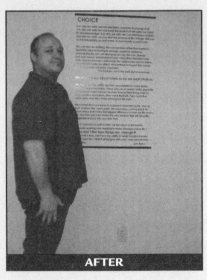

BEFORE   **AFTER**

I have spent a lifetime attempting to control my weight. Having an Italian background has not helped—food was used as a reward for just about everything. I attempted just about every method I could research to lose the weight, including starvation. I would lose some weight but could never keep it off.

As I grew, so did my waistline, but with every failed attempt at weight loss I fell deeper into denial, until I accepted that I would always be a fat man. It wasn't long before I simply stopped trying to lose the weight, and I began to get exponentially heavier as the years passed. My health began to deteriorate; I was unable to do the simplest of tasks—tie my shoes or even put my own socks on. My poor wife had to complete these tasks for me. Doctor visits became rare, as I was too embarrassed and afraid of seeing a doctor, but I had eventually developed conditions that required medication to control my blood sugar, blood pressure, cholesterol, and sleep apnea. I convinced myself that it was all genetic.

I did nothing but gain weight throughout my twenties. I had a terrific job that was full of opportunity, and I continually saw people advancing. Although I had all the tools and had proven that I was more effective than several other individuals who had advanced, I was continually overlooked; this added to my depression and I began to eat more to comfort myself.

The V.P. of the company I worked for had successfully lost 30 pounds with Harvey's help; he asked me to come to one of the Sunday classes. I avoided the situation, because I felt that I was beyond help.

But three weeks later I found myself walking into Harvey's place, still panting from the stair climb. I had no idea what I weighed; I never had a desire to find out how heavy I really was. I walked into this program a five-foot-nine 39-year-old man who weighed 461 pounds. I listened to Harvey speak, and it was very good therapy; I could relate to a lot of what the other members were experiencing—but I still did not think that this would work for me. I listened to the CDs and followed the program, which was surprisingly easy to understand and follow, and returned the following Sunday for the weigh-in. I had lost seven pounds that week.

It was not a diet; it was a new beginning, a new way of eating and a new way of living, and I loved it. Today I'm medication-free, with a clean bill of health. I'm 190 pounds lighter, with a new job promotion.

Harvey has improved my health, helped me regain my confidence and brought me closer to my family and children. He has given me the opportunity to spend many more years enjoying the life that I once thought was empty and futile. Harvey has saved my life.

Louie D'Arpino

This chapter deals with the most direct effects that obesity has on three distinct areas of your day-to-day existence. You need to understand that if you continue to gain weight, and don't get back to (and maintain) a proper weight, you're ruining your life. Your own anxiety may have led you towards being overweight. This causes lowered self-esteem because it has negative consequences for three extremely important areas of your life: your health, your career, and your sex life.

I didn't write this book to make men appear stupid. After all, I'm a man, and I still remember all the bitter personal experiences from my own obesity crisis. However, I've concluded—after years of self-examination, and working with thousands of men—that when it comes to an understanding of what affects their weight and how weight affects their life, men (including me) have traditionally been woefully naïve.

If you're like me, you're slow to change your ways. So if I'm going to help you then I've got to provide some very graphic examples of where you are headed, or, in some cases, where you already are today.

Pause a moment, and think about how you feel both physically and emotionally. I want you to burn this feeling that you have at this moment into your very soul. It's important to do this, because when I get you back to the top of the fitness hill, you'll need to be able to draw on this feeling and use it as personal motivation. I'm going to make sure that you never slide down into this gully again.

YOU'RE OVERWEIGHT AND YOU EXPECT TO REMAIN HEALTHY?

Men are usually dismissive of health issues, and rarely visit a doctor until they are very sick. When we do visit the doctor, we're usually given the same advice: "You've got to lose 30 pounds." Wanting to please him or her, we dutifully ask, "How?" If we're lucky we get a brochure with some tips. Sometimes the doctor will recommend seeing a nutritionist, or that we start walking or working out. And maybe we give it a passing try for a few days, but we don't stick with it, because we haven't understood that it's not a temporary effort. *You can't lose weight and then go back to old habits.* Losing weight permanently demands a life change, which is why I call my program the ONE**80** plan: it's going to turn your life around. Unfortunately, to make this kind of turn around, we need more advice and support than a doctor can provide in that short time.

What usually happens is that we go back to the status quo, and we continue to gain weight and lose our health. At the next medical exam, the doctor again identifies one or more of the following symptoms: high blood sugar levels, high cholesterol levels, and high blood pressure—warning signs of diseases associated with being overweight. This time your doctor's response is stronger: "You've got to lose weight, or your life will be at risk!"

Now if we were sane, this message would motivate us. We're not, and it doesn't. I've talked to the doctors and to the patients who received the message. On the next visit, if things have continued to get worse and your life is now seriously at risk, your doctor is forced to prescribe drugs to control the various problems that are arising from your eating habits. If you're religious about taking your drugs, they slow the onslaught of health problems. But you're drug-dependent now, you're not healthy, and you're still gaining weight. Inevitably, you're going to need more drugs, and you're going to be risking those nasty side affects that form the last 20 seconds of every drug advertisement. Worse yet, you have no idea how the various drugs that you're taking will react with each other. You're certainly not solving your problem.

I recently asked a new client if he had any health issues. His answer was that he was in "great health." His only problem was that he was overweight. I decided to press him, and he went on to tell me that he had diabetes, high blood pressure, and high cholesterol, but "they're all being managed by medication." It's amazing how we can delude ourselves. Clearly it's the medications that are keeping him alive. How foolish and delusional we men can be!

STATISTICS LINK SERIOUS DISEASES TO BEING OVERWEIGHT

Becoming overweight or obese is an ever-growing health curse, and it's costing our societies literally billions of dollars. In North America alone, obesity causes over 300,000 premature deaths each year. It is second only to smoking as the leading cause of preventable death. Since 2001, countless articles have been published on the issue, and yet, despite constant warnings in the media, many men remain unaware of the serious risks associated with not managing their weight. Men are between 25 and 33 percent more likely to get colon, rectum, prostate, esophageal, and kidney cancer if they are obese. About 70 percent of cardiovascular disease can be traced to obesity, and 90 percent of type 2 diabetics are overweight.

We've got to ask ourselves: what's wrong with us? When there are recurring news articles on how our existing diets are killing us, why are we continuing to eat the same way? Of course, we all know the answer. We don't believe that anything will happen to *us*. Statistics are about other people. Right? Wrong!

Men don't tend to believe that the physical problems they experience are attached to their eating habits. However, according to WebMD—whose material is vetted by the Cleveland Clinic—a man who is 40 percent above his appropriate weight is twice as likely to die prematurely as is his average-weight male neighbor. This is because a man's physiology is not meant to store significant amounts of fat and if it's accumulated, it can be incredibly dangerous.

MEN AND WOMEN ARE DIFFERENT WHEN IT COMES TO EXCESS WEIGHT

Of course, it isn't healthy for anyone to become obese or to carry around too much extra fat. However, women are genetically able and predisposed to store some fat, because they need to build up reserves to support a baby when they become pregnant, and to breastfeed afterward. They tend to put the weight on around their hips, thighs, and buttocks, where it does them little harm even if they don't lose it later in life. In fact, recent medical literature suggests some fat is actually good for them as they move into menopause. People who store fat around the thighs and hips are commonly referred to as "pear-shaped."

Men, on the other hand, tend to become "apple-shaped": they put weight on around the waist. This so-called spare tire poses a very significant health hazard. Men whose weight is concentrated like this are at greater risk of developing heart disease, diabetes, or cancer than overweight women. Visceral fat located in the stomach area also affects organs such as the heart and lungs. For example, a waist circumference of 36 inches is associated with a high-risk profile for coronary heart disease.

IF YOU'RE AN OVERWEIGHT MAN, YOU CAN'T POSSIBLY BE FEELING WELL!

You may be reading this section, and saying to yourself that you actually feel all right . . . and I'm here to tell you that you've forgotten what feeling "well" really means. The number one reason men show up at my clinic is because they feel awful and they've been sent by a friend or their doctor. They're taking all kinds of medications and want to get off them. You'll know this from reading some of the testimonials at the beginning of each chapter.

Can Hardly Walk #1: "My Joints Are Killing Me!"

When you are carrying extra pounds, you place extra pressure on your knee, hip, and lower back joints. This pressure gradually wears away the cartilage (the tissue that cushions the joints) that normally protects them, in a condition called osteoarthritis. The more these joints are bothering you, the less likely you are to be physically active. So you burn fewer calories throughout the day and maintain less muscle mass. Because muscles burn more calories than fat, as you lose your muscle mass you'll see even more weight gain. Eventually your knee or hip will need to be replaced. You can see that it becomes a vicious circle and will inevitably lead to other medical problems. The good news is that weight loss can decrease stress on the knees, hips, and lower back and may improve the symptoms of osteoarthritis. If you manage your food intake first, it won't be long before you can start to up your exercise.

Can Hardly Walk #2: "There's Nothing More Painful Than Gout in Your Big Toe."

Gout is a disease that affects the joints. It is caused by high levels of a substance called uric acid in the blood; it can form solid or crystal-like masses that deposit in the joints, often in your foot. The consequences can be swelling (to the point where you can't put on your shoe) and excruciating pain. Gout is often an inherited condition, so if you know of a family member who has suffered with it, you are at greater risk. Regardless of your family's medical history, you are more likely to develop gout if you are overweight, and the more overweight you are, the higher the risk.

Another Way That Being Overweight Can Cause Serious Pain

Ask any friend who's had a gallstone—it's a very big ouch! Guess what: gallbladder disease and gallstones are more common if you are overweight, and the risk of disease increases as your weight increases. While the cause is not clear, you must be very careful if you have this problem. Rapid weight loss, or losing a lot of weight, can actually increase your chances of redeveloping gallstones. Doctors recommend modest, *slow* weight loss—usually around two or three pounds per week, depending on how much you need to lose.

Non-Deadly Misery #1: Heartburn

Practically every overweight man I meet suffers from severe heartburn (acid indigestion). They'll tell me that they need to swallow antacid pills by the handful to cure the pain. I understand that in its worst form, it can feel like a heart attack. If this is a condition that you suffer from, you should know that a change in your diet can be your cure. When you start eating properly, this is a symptom that can and will go away.

Non-Deadly Misery #2: Sleep Apnea

Arthur was another client, a 52-year-old accountant. While he had been gaining some weight, he thought that he was going along fine. Then he noticed that in only one year he had gained 15 pounds. Being a numbers guy, he did the calculations on how much he would weigh if this progression kept up. He was already developing a serious health problem, and knew that things were going to get worse in a hurry. He was on a prescription for cholesterol pills, but what was really bothering him was his sleep apnea.

"My wife told me that I stopped breathing in the middle of the night. She said that the snoring that resulted was keeping her and my daughter awake and that they couldn't continue to go through this. I didn't know what sleep apnea was."

Sleep apnea is a serious breathing condition associated with being overweight. It develops because overweight men build up fatty deposits around vital organs and in the muscles around the throat; when they go to sleep, those muscles relax, the throat closes, and they stop breathing. This causes them to briefly black out because of lack of oxygen. The brain realizes the problem and pumps a large dose of adrenalin to jolt them awake and get them going again. That causes the snoring gasp that your sleep partner may have described to you. This process can happen up to 200 times per hour.

It will cause a man to snore heavily, and it can also cause daytime sleepiness and even lead to heart failure. The risk for sleep apnea increases as body weight increases. Weight loss usually improves sleep apnea.

In Arthur's case, he went for the test. "You sleep with a mask all night and with stuff on your fingers to measure the blood flow. To my shock, I discovered that I was waking up 118 times per hour. This situation could have resulted in me dying of a heart attack!" This is because

Arthur's blood pressure would go way up when his brain was not getting enough oxygen. (In essence, there wasn't enough oxygen getting into the blood, and so the heart had to pump harder.) Unfortunately, Arthur's initial reaction was to do what so many other men choose: ignore the real reason behind his sleep apnea and use a machine to deal with his problems. These continuous positive air pressure (CPAP) machines pump oxygen and cost about $1,200. Around 70 percent of them are being sold to obese men. With the apnea machine and a humidifier, men with the ailment can sleep sort of normally. (Arthur described trying to travel with all this equipment: "Just think of my hassles going through security, not to mention the lifting associated with the equipment.")

Again, the good news ending: Arthur lost the weight, and his sleep apnea and the CPAP machine went away. "When you stop snoring, you can't believe how grateful your wife can be."

Slow Death: Increased Risk of Diabetes

Diabetes means that your body can't control the sugar levels in your blood stream. Type 2 diabetes usually occurs later in a man's life and is generally associated with being overweight. (In fact, being overweight makes a man almost twice as likely to develop the disease.) Diabetes is a major cause of early death, heart disease, stroke, and blindness. The good news is that if you've developed the disease, losing weight and be coming more physically active can help control your blood sugar levels and may allow you to reduce the amount of medication that you need.

Sudden Death: Heart Disease and Stroke

Overweight men are twice as likely to have high blood pressure, a major risk factor for heart disease and stroke, than men who are not overweight. In addition, very high levels of HDL cholesterol in the blood are often linked to being overweight and can also lead to heart disease. Heart disease and stroke are the leading causes of death and disability (without any signs or symptoms) for people in North America. Being overweight also contributes to angina, which is chest pain caused by decreased oxygen to the heart.

The good news is that losing a small amount of weight can reduce your chances of developing heart disease or having a stroke. Reducing your weight by 10 percent can decrease your chance of developing heart disease.

A Man's Diet and Cancer

My theory is that if you're an overweight man, you've been eating an inappropriate diet for a long time. You've been filling yourself with fast food, processed food, and food that generally contains too much fat and sugar, and far too many calories. While the direct links are still being investigated, it seems that overweight men are at higher risk for developing colorectal cancer and prostate cancer. To me, it doesn't matter whether the increased risk is due to the extra weight or to a high-fat, high-calorie diet. It's not a risk that a sane individual would want to take. It is time to make a permanent change with regard to what you're going to put in your body. The effects are reversible if men achieve and maintain a lower weight.

YOU'RE OVERWEIGHT AND YOU EXPECT TO MAXIMIZE YOUR SUCCESS IN YOUR CAREER?

Research confirms that "size still matters" . . . and I don't mean it the way you are thinking! Overweight men are judged more harshly at work. Employers judge an overweight man as someone who is not in control. His appearance and clothes speak of his low self-esteem. This is not a man who gives off the vibes of success. Your employer, staff, colleagues, and clients, though they may not admit it, are strongly affected by the way you present yourself.

Job Prospects Can Become Limited

Ask yourself this question: "If two equally smart and qualified men apply for the same job, and one is overweight and one is not, who is more likely to be the successful candidate?" If your answer is the trim guy, then I think that you'd be right over 90 percent of the time. It's an unhappy fact, but in fairness to the potential employer, there are reasons why they come to this conclusion.

If you're the heavy guy, when you eliminate the excess weight, you take away those concerns and bias (justified or unjustified). Being a trim and healthy man will give you the confidence and the energy to compete successfully for years to come!

Your Weight and Health Costs

As we've discussed, being overweight has a very direct affect on the chances that you will be afflicted with a serious ailment. Your employers know this as well as you do. There are two specific ways your being overweight will affect them. The first is absenteeism. They look at you, and they have the statistical proof that you will miss work for health reasons more often than your trim coworkers. When you're away from the job, your employer needs to find someone to replace you. This costs them in dollars spent and productivity, because your replacement is not going to be able to do your job as well as you do. As a result, the company is faced with overtime, or even more temporary help. If you're in the service business, they also risk unhappy clients.

The other cost to your employer comes from increased insurance premiums for the company. The more you use the health care system, the more it costs. An employer who hires you has to anticipate taking on a greater cost than if he or she hires someone who does not have a weight problem. This is why so many companies today are providing cash bonuses for those who are willing to lose weight.

Does Your Weight Leave You with the Energy to Do the Job?

Manny was a design development manager for a home building company. Describing his relationship with me, he says, "When I met Harvey, I was just short of 300 pounds on a 5-foot-8-inch frame. I felt sluggish every day, and I was beginning to know that I would be unable to keep what I had, let alone move farther ahead. Fortunately, I had several discussions with my employer where he reiterated that I had to do something. He opened up a gym downstairs and with the advice from Harvey and the support of the office, I lost 85 pounds and got my life back on track. I always say that 'yesterday's performance is why you can come to work tomorrow,' and I'm getting in shape so that I'll be able to do what's necessary to have the energy to be competitive over the next 10 to 15 years."

Alfred was a 44-year-old civil engineer and part-time accountant who came into my practice. When he first arrived, he weighed 480 pounds. "I was a senior inspector and personally didn't feel productive . . . I just didn't feel like doing it. In retrospect, I didn't have the energy. While I did a good job on the places that I did manage to inspect, I knew that I was short-changing my company. Through my work with Harvey, I've now reduced my weight to 225 pounds. Today, I feel totally different. I've now had three job offers from other towns and cities. Now life is definitely on the up and up."

It's not just physical jobs where energy matters. Seymour is a 65-year-old lawyer who was attending my program and lost 40 pounds. "I spend long hours at my office, and work better now than seven years ago. I no longer get tired, and the day goes by more quickly. Energy is no longer a concern."

Do Overweight Guys Reach the Top of the Heap?

During all my time working with men, I've noticed that very few CEOs are fat. In fact, I've had men come to my class who realized that they could be in line for a promotion and wanted to do something about their weight before the moment of truth arrived. Not everyone is destined to be a CEO, but pretty much everyone is destined to work, and we'd all like to advance in our jobs. If you're like most of the men I know, then you're hoping that you'll be maximizing your return for those hours that you're spending at work. I know that you will only do this if you have high self-esteem and are making the best possible impression with your colleagues.

Can Overweight Guys Be Successful Entrepreneurs?

The easy answer is yes, and there are lots of examples. However, I've coached a lot of entrepreneurs in my time and they've told me of times when they've been moving rapidly towards a deal on the phone, and then seen the brakes applied when they met the other party for the first time. They've wondered if the person was secretly thinking, "Do I really want to do business with this guy?" Of course, if the deal falls apart, they never know the real reason. Given the competitive world they occupy, they've said to me that they never want to take that chance again.

What Does a Fat You Reflect on Your Company?

A client of mine called Steve sells residential homes. He had been married three times, and when he was going through the break-ups, he would bury his emotions in food. He says, "There's no question that it affected business; people don't want a fat guy showing them property. You could see the disappointment in their eyes. Even the people who would come back and talk to me were looking at my stomach. There were areas, like the attic, where I couldn't go because I literally didn't fit. I really felt very self-conscious." The good news is that after working with me Steve has now lost 45 pounds and is maintaining a consistent weight. Now that he is again full of energy and has high self-esteem, he's found that he's enjoying life more and his clients want to be around him again.

He Thinks More about Food Than He Does about Work!

If you've gained this much weight, then the chances are good that you spend a great deal of time thinking about the next time you eat. It's not likely that you are the type of man who will work through lunch or a coffee break. Your managers know this, and while there's nothing wrong with taking some time from work, I know that it makes them anxious. If you're bringing food to your desk and worrying about how to keep yourself satisfied, then over a year, you're spending a lot of work hours worrying about your food rather than your job. This is certainly not the summary that you want on your annual review or your resume.

YOU'RE OVERWEIGHT AND YOU EXPECT AN ACTIVE SEX LIFE?

I know that this is a tough part of your life to confront, but I want you to be honest with yourself and ask yourself what has happened to your sexuality, sensuality, and intimacy since you've been gaining weight. After you've read this section, ask yourself if you haven't been ignoring the fact that a number of these circumstances are a real part of life for you and your partner.

Sex and Self-Esteem

One of the first issues to think about in regard to your sex life is self-esteem. A great sex life can only be developed with a person who is comfortable and confident in his own body. If you're really overweight, it's my bet that a great deal of that positive self-image has been lost, along with the ability to be a really great lover. If you're asking your partner to make compromises in bed because of your weight, then you're not being as good a partner as you might have once been. If that's happening, then it is likely to result in your sex life deteriorating, and this in turn will cause you to have lower self-esteem. It's a vicious cycle that can only be reversed in one way. Eat right and think about how much greater your confidence would be in your retrofitted body. Makes you want to take it for a test drive, doesn't it?

No Sex and Lack of Self-Esteem

If you're fit, and you maintain a balanced and satisfying sex life into your sixties and later, then that fact alone goes a long way to relieving stress and helping keep your relationship happy. I can attest to this because it's worked for Helen and me. However, if because of your weight your sex life has suffered or ceased to exist, then the chances are good that you're now adding stress to your life, and this stress is not going to be relieved by being intimate. Instead, chances are good that this stress is being relieved by eating, and so you are perpetuating the vicious cycle, which results in an even greater lack of self-esteem. This is obviously not healthy for you as an individual, but it can be very destructive if you are in a relationship. Issues that are no longer softened by a good sexual relationship build up as a means of covering for the "unspoken" problem that is becoming beyond repair.

Sex and Performance

Your self-esteem may be strong enough to permit you to remain a good lover when you are overweight, but there's another very serious problem. The greater your weight, the farther your blood must circulate. Your erection depends on a strong supply of blood to your penis. If your heart is strained by having to move your blood much farther through a much larger body, then, you guessed it: you're going to experience problems getting and maintaining an erection. In effect, the mind may be willing, but the body will say no!

Sex and Your Penis

Let's just say that you're really lucky and that you have a great heart and great circulation even though you are overweight. There's another problem that you will notice if you look over that belly that you've created. You may be surprised to learn that fat is stored everywhere, including the area around the penis. More weight stretches the skin of the abdomen, and draws the penis in, making it both shorter and smaller. It's one thing to be able to put up with the embarrassment (but who wants to?) when you are showering with other men, but here comes a far worse reality. The next time that you want to have sex with your partner, you may get your erection all right, but it will be one that is a rather poor replica of what you could produce when you were at your proper weight. This affects your self-esteem and your relationship, and all the positive thoughts in the world can't change it.

Sex and Your Partner

A lovely woman who was married to an overweight man told me that her sex life was adversely affected because she was constantly worried about being, as she said, "squished." Who's going to want to be in bed with a guy who could slip off his elbows and push all the air out of his partner's lungs? It's just not a romantic thought!

Sexual Positions

I suppose that this is another example of the obvious! If variety is the spice of life, then it's safe to say that you're going to be rather limited in your spice rack if you've allowed yourself to become significantly overweight. You'll be spending most if not all of your nights lying on your back, because after a while, no other position works.

Sex and Fitness

There are some issues associated with sex that are just common sense, but you may not have thought of them. The most obvious is that good sex requires energy, right? And if you're out of shape, you're also going to be out of energy in a hurry. Add to that endless nights snoring and no sleep (for both of you) . . . that's not going to make for great performance.

Sex and Your Libido

One of the most significant issues is that gaining weight lowers your libido. It can get so bad that you don't care whether or not you have sex. One of my clients, Jules, a 44-year old dentist, expressed his feelings very clearly: "Sex is the last thing on your mind; everything is in the way." Interestingly, this is a uniquely male problem that does not affect women, whose hormones are different. As for Jules, he has now lost 150 pounds—and how things have changed.

Sex and Procreation

If you're young and hoping to have a family, then losing your interest is not a good thing. However, even if your libido survives and you are having sex, you are producing less sperm! Obviously, if you have less sperm, there is less chance of conception. The good news is that losing that weight can help you with your fertility.

Sex on Your Own

Maybe you're thinking to yourself, it's all too complicated. If I can't find a partner who loves me for what I am, then I can always masturbate. Well, even masturbation gets more and more difficult. Like intercourse, masturbation takes energy, and if you continue the way you're going, you will have less of it each year. You're also going to be faced with reaching around that massive gut to touch an ever-smaller penis. It's not a great prognosis, but I'm hitting you with it, so that you'll be motivated to reverse the weight gaining trend and get back to your old self!

Improved Sex after Weight Loss

The good news is that duration and frequency of sex can and will increase after you lose weight, and you'll find some very happy case histories throughout this book to help prove the point.

I think that you're beginning to get the picture. Being overweight has very real negative effects on your physical health, your employment prospects, and your intimate relationships. Dealing with incredible stress in these three critical areas of your life can make having healthy self-esteem seem as possible as a trip to the moon. But the great news is that focusing on your diet and taking control of your body will have an equally positive effect on each of these key areas of your life. The confidence that comes from knowing that you're not only healthy but also looking great will have an immediate positive effect on your work and your relationships. It's simple. You got yourself into this situation, and with the right tools and some well-earned support, you're perfectly capable of getting yourself out of it.

THE DIET INDUSTRY IS AN UNREGULATED SCAM

5

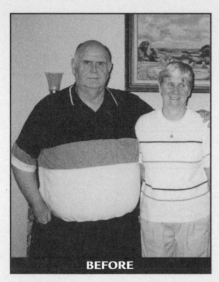

BEFORE

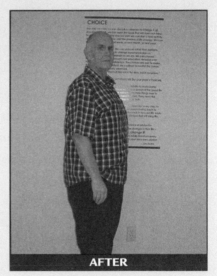

AFTER

I have been big my entire life. In 1971 I got married and weighed 229 pounds. I gained weight afterwards, and by November 2004 I weighed 349 pounds. I joined Harvey Brooker's group and have learned so much from him and my fellow classmates. One word: education.

Before attending Harvey's classes I didn't pay attention to product labels. If I wanted something, I bought it and ate it. I no longer do that. Thanks to Harvey I now read and understand labels and this has made a considerable difference. I now know what I'm eating and am much healthier than ever before.

My weight loss is now 122 pounds, which puts me below my weight in 1971, and that's what I wanted to do. It is because of Harvey Brooker and his words of wisdom that I was able to lose the weight and now understand how to keep it off and be healthy for the rest of my life.

Don Oates

During my 20-plus years of counseling men from every walk of life, hundreds have come to me for help after being unsuccessful with diet programs. I understand the temptation to search for the simple solution, and I've made it part of my life's work to keep up with each new offer as it's presented to the public. I analyze the fad diets. I've heard countless heartbreaking stories that result from the get-thin-quick schemes. I've had doctors explain the chemistry behind those diets that feature certain food products to temporarily trick your body into losing weight (often water or muscle loss). I share these stories with you so that you can develop a critical eye, which will help you judge new programs as they jump out at you from the media.

First off, promise yourself that even if you chose not to follow the direction in this book, you will never again be sucked in to the foolishness that most people are buying. Ignore the impossible promises (10 pounds in 10 days!), and ask yourself, Who do you know personally who has lost weight permanently on any of these programs?

I call the weight loss industry "the potions and lotions business." It's worth $58 billion and growing each year in the United States. What a great industry—the only one in the world whose continuous failure guarantees its geometric growth and success. It works, because people lose weight, gain it back, and need to diet again. Dieters are a never-ending source of income for those who have figured out how to profit from our unfortunate eating habits. There's lots of competition, but what a great place to be an executive.

Yes, there are some first-rate individuals and institutions that are breaking new ground while trying to contribute to a positive change. However, as the industry is completely unregulated, they are more often drowned out by the clamor of the scam artists trying to siphon your hard-earned money from your wallet.

Promises, promises, and more promises. It's not easy to govern the soothsayers and charlatans, be they lay people or medical people, when it comes to selling the prospect of losing weight. Most overweight men would sell their soul to the devil, if only the devil would show them a quick path to Thinsville.

In the world of the circus, a good metaphor for dieting, one of P.T. Barnum's competitors, while watching crowds form for a Barnum show noted, "There's a sucker born every minute." Nowhere is that more true than in the hungry mind of an overweight person willing to try or buy anything, "if this fat will just go away!" It's ironic, given the amount of fat and sugar in much of the food that we eat, that getting money for diet products truly is like taking candy from a baby.

Where else in the business world could an industry get away with removing billions of dollars in just the United States and Canada and have no lasting tangible results? (At least P.T. Barnum gave them a show.)

Maybe you're saying to yourself, "Why is Harvey's eating program different?" My program is guided by three principles:

1. Your food has to be nutritionally sound.
2. Your food has to be portable, so that you can stick to the program anywhere.
3. Your food should leave you feeling satisfied and never hungry.

Those principles probably appeal to your common sense, and, as you will soon see, you'll be spending your money where you should be: at the grocery store.

I think that when you've taken the time to read this book, you'll accept that there's nothing magical in what I'm saying. My program comes down to teaching your male body and mind to work hard to change your lifetime eating habits. To lose one pound of fat you must achieve a deficit of 3,500 calories. I'm going to show you an easy way of doing this which will never allow you to feel famished. I'll also provide you with my experience on why there is so rarely any lasting effect from various other diet programs.

ANY DIET THAT DOES NOT LET YOU EAT NORMAL (GROCERY-BOUGHT) FOOD WON'T WORK

Diets do not work on a permanent basis because they are not permanent life changes. Sure you've seen some before-and-after shots of so-called successful clients, but how come we never see the successful five-years-after photos? Answer: they don't exist! Fully 99 percent of men who go on a diet have gained over 100 percent of their weight back within two years. Diets are by nature unsustainable; you don't need to go on a special diet. You need the knowledge and support of a dedicated professional who can help you create a lifelong program that works.

Avoid Miracle Cure Diets

These diets all claim to have discovered a magic chemical that will cause your body to lose weight. These diets usually revolve around a product that you can get only from that company. So are you going to take these supplements for a lifetime? What about the rest of your lifestyle and eating habits? Is anyone coaching you? While the magic potion is important for the profits of the company, it is most often irrelevant to successful weight loss, or even detrimental! Magic potions can be pills, they can be injections, and they can be drinks that purport to have all the nutrition that you need in a day. Many of them can seem to work at first. None can work for a lifetime.

Avoid the Boxed Food Brigade

These diets also work while you're on them because you're essentially paying a company to measure and send you appropriate helpings. The company earns exorbitant profits by charging a premium for packaging and sending you food that you could purchase in your neighborhood grocery store. They do not teach you how to make these foods yourself. Ask yourself if you're going to eat nothing but pre-packaged food for the rest of your life, and if the answer is no, then you can understand why this kind of a program will not work in the long run.

Avoid the "All Natural" Diet

The next is the "natural" diet, where the "expert" asks us to look to our ancient ancestors and the natural world for the answer. With the world's move to green, it is popular to associate the word *natural* with healthy foods and with many weight loss products. However, just because products are made from natural ingredients or ingredients that have been around for an eternity, doesn't mean they are effective, or safe.

Megan Ogilvie, health writer for the *Toronto Star*, notes: "Many of the active ingredients in over-the-counter weight loss supplements are derived from plants, minerals and other natural sources . . . Although many people assume natural means safe, the products can have drug-like properties and cause serious health problems. But unlike pharmaceuticals, natural weight loss remedies don't have to go through rigorous clinical trials."

The fact is that there are few effective regulations on over-the-counter products sold for weight loss in either Canada or the United States. In her article, Ogilvie goes on to cite a 2004 study by Robert Saper, director of integrative medicine at Boston University Medical Center. He found that "none of the 26 most common ingredients in over-the-counter weight loss supplements, including green tea, chromium, and guar gum, met acceptable criteria for safety and efficacy." He also said companies "skirted the ephedra ban by using related chemicals, such as those found in bitter orange plants, which can also cause cardiovascular problems."

Saper has since turned his attention to analyzing active ingredients in "natural" weight loss supplements. Right now, he says, many of the products imported into North America contain impurities, such as pesticides and heavy metals, or are adulterated with prescription drugs.

Avoid the Eat-the-Same-and-Take-This-Pill Diet

We can always look to the pharmaceutical professionals to come up with another diet pill. At the moment there are prescription weight loss drugs such as Meridia™ and the generic phentermine, which make you feel full, suppress cravings, or curb your appetite. As I will discuss later, you can do this just as well by choosing regular grocery store food, without any of the nasty side effects and without becoming drug-dependent.

There are also pills that block your absorption of fat. Writing in the *Wall Street Journal* on July 19, 2007, Tara Parker-Pope reviewed the new nonprescription diet drug Alli™ as "flying off the store shelves." However, she went on to say that "most people who use it will lose very little weight and may experience embarrassing side effects." Alli, produced by GlaxoSmithKline, is the first of these over-the-counter drugs to win FDA approval. It prevents the body from breaking down fat and absorbing it. Alli is supposed to block about 25 percent of the fat that you eat. Parker-Pope's article states that one in five people using the drug will lose 10 percent of their body weight, and half will lose five percent of their body weight. The product, which is to be taken with meals, also has its downside. Tara Parker-Pope humorously quotes the Glaxo website, myalli.com, which warns the drug can cause gas with oily discharge as well as frequent or loose stools. The site suggests it's probably "a smart idea" to wear dark pants and bring a change of clothes to work if you use Alli!

Avoid the Food Group Diet

The next is the "one kind of food" diet. They are all different, and yet all the same: don't eat carbs, don't eat fat, only eat protein—you name it; they'll have you trying it. The problems with these diets are innumerable, but the most important issue is that we need all three of our macronutrients (carbohydrates, fats, and proteins) to stay alive and to stay healthy. Any diet that tries to cut one out is dead wrong from the outset and will cause your body harm.

Avoid the Weight Loss Resorts

There are spas and weight loss resorts that are legitimately helping people by training them to eat healthier and exercise appropriately. They usually cost $5,000 or more per week, which makes even a single week impossible for most people. For those who can afford the time and cost, these spas and resorts can work for a time. Trouble is, you've got to go home sooner or later. I'll give you a famous example.

You may remember baseball umpire John McSherry, who died on opening day of the 1996 baseball season. He was in Cincinnati, behind home plate. During the first inning he turned to the home plate camera, waved time out, took off his mask, and fell to his knees. He died, right there in front of millions on TV and a packed stadium. The baseball world and its fans were stunned.

To my recollection, all the reports on TV and in newspaper articles said something like "McSherry dies of heart attack"—except for one periodical, the *Baseball News*, which reported correctly that McSherry had died from obesity, which caused his heart attack.

As a result of his early death, Eric Gregg, another very overweight umpire and a friend of McSherry's, took a leave of absence from Major League Baseball to enter a weight reduction program at Duke University where he lost approximately 60 pounds. In his recent eulogy—he died at 55—it was said that he had lost some weight after John McSherry's death, but that he regained it after coming home from the weight loss facility.

So unless you've got unlimited funds and unlimited time and can afford to be away from your work and your family, you'd be better off learning how to eat well all of the time, in any situation. Save your holiday time for just that—holidays.

Avoid the Group Programs Aimed Only at Women

When a program is aimed at women, the group leader is usually a woman who has lost weight on that system, and the clientele and the issues discussed are normally dominated by women. Most men find the novelty of being the only man in the room quickly wears thin. Women are different physiologically. They lose weight differently. Things that motivate women in a group usually don't motivate men. I believe that men are more responsive to male leaders and that women are more responsive to female leaders because it's easier to talk openly about issues and motivation with someone of your own sex.

Even more important, the eating program must be both disciplined, and based on keeping a man feeling full. Eating programs for women rarely appeal to men, and in some cases even allow them to bank points that let them cheat on the program. In my observation any "cheat," whether it's "legal" or not, leads you inevitably back to square one. A parallel to saving points for a legal cheat would be an alcoholic's saying, "Well, I've been good all week, so I owe myself." It can't work. It's never worked. You may already know this because you've been on diets that have failed you by sabotaging your efforts and undermining your determination.

Avoid Laparoscopic Surgery

This surgery can be a permanent solution, but it is by far the most dangerous solution, and it doesn't leave much room for a normal life. It forces you to eat bird-sized potions of food, having already faced all the risks that are associated with any kind of surgery. Recently on local TV, I saw a patient and the bariatric surgeon who had performed his procedure. The doctor admitted that when the patient went to a buffet with his family, his stomach size meant he had to chew and then spit out his food. Does a sane individual actually feel that this is the better way?

Avoid the "Doctor Solution"

A surprising number of men will go through a period of total despair—they give up on getting healthy altogether, and decide to rely on their doctor to keep them going. The problem is that doctors can't manage men's eating; they can only manage the results. As they don't have the time or training to treat the causes of male obesity, they treat the symptoms instead, with high blood pressure pills or cholesterol reducing pills. These medications temporarily mask a symptom, but your weight will still creep up, and your health will still deteriorate.

By now you must be thinking, "If the pills, boxed food, weight loss stores, lose-weight-while-you-sleep, high-protein, low-protein, cabbage soup, Miami Diet, Hollywood diet, this doctor's and that doctor's diets all fail, then tell me: what does work?"

My program works. It works for men. I'm not asking you to starve yourself, or take pills, or get shots. I'm not going to cut back on a major food group, or try to entice you with one-food wonder diets. I'm not going to tell you to eat seven times a day, or to skip lunch, or to have breakfast for dinner, or that deep breathing while you eat will instantly cause 20 pounds to disappear from your gut. I am going to show you a no-nonsense program that involves regular portions of regular foods. I am also going to show you that you can be motivated to positively change how you eat and think about yourself, and that if you change how you eat in a way that will never leave you hungry, you will be able to do that for the rest of your life.

Luckily, in anything we wish to accomplish, there are professionals who are able to pass on their experience to students or clients who wish to learn what is being taught. There are law professors to teach law; there are piano teachers to teach piano. Every skill and every trade has knowledgeable people in the forefront who can teach, mentor, or coach others.

And learning a healthy way to attain your appropriate weight and maintain it for a lifetime is like anything else: learning from a dedicated professional is the way to success.

You might be saying to yourself that you learn from experience. But look at your own life and where you are today, especially if you have tried a number of weight loss methods without success. Here's my take on experience: it's a terrible teacher—you get the test first and the lesson afterwards. My ambition with this book is to become the mentor that you need to take you from your first dropped pound to a lifetime of maintaining a healthy weight.

I have spent 35 years learning what works and what doesn't for men. I've written this book for the man who wants the long truth rather than the short lie, so he can get on with his life. I teach this to the 150 or so men who gather to hear me speak each week and in the one-to-one coaching I perform both in person and over the phone in the United States and Canada. I can show any man how to be free of this demeaning, self-esteem-destroying, health-threatening situation.

For once and forever—with no pain, no hunger, no gimmicks, no special foods to buy, just good old common sense and a healthy eating program that's full of great food choices—you really can lose the weight and get back to your old self. You can lose weight the same way you gained it . . . with a knife and fork.

Let's move on and find out exactly how my program works.

PART 2

THE ONE80 PLAN

MAKE CHANGE
YOUR PROJECT

6

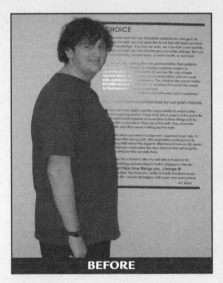

BEFORE

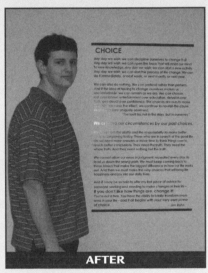

AFTER

As my seventeenth birthday was approaching, I had all but given up on the idea that I would lose weight. At 276 pounds, I was unattractive, unhealthy, and completely out of control. Finally I decided that enough was enough and joined the Harvey Brooker Weight Loss Program. While I had occasionally tried to control my eating before, I had never been successful for long. Yet this was different. Harvey's program wasn't like the gimmicks sold on TV. It was just a common-sense program to eat less food and make sure that the foods that I did eat were healthy.

Make no mistake: there's no magic, easy way of losing weight. While following Harvey's program gives you the tools you need, there's only one person who can lose your weight, and that's you. It's not an easy process. My weight loss required constant vigilance and was fraught with hurdles. It meant writing down everything that I put into my mouth, and saying no to fatty or sugary confections—even to one bite. It also meant having faith in myself and never giving up, no matter what obstacles were in my way.

Making the decision to start living a healthy life seems like it would be an easy one, but it is not. This isn't a temporary plan just to shed weight and go back to the way you were eating before. Joining this program means completely rejecting the life you are living now. It means telling yourself that you will never again have that basket of fries, or piece of chocolate cake, or fatty restaurant pizza. Not in a month, not in a year, and not in a decade. If you aren't willing to make that kind of permanent sacrifice, then your efforts will only be met with failure. But if you've finally decided that you've had enough with always being that fat guy, like I did, and you're willing to put in the work to change the way you live, then I assure you that you will never look back. One year later and 60 pounds lighter, I know that I never have.

Kevin Wiener

Few men have the stamina to embrace change and stay with it. Those who do so deserve to be singled out as men among men. I want you to be one of them. I hope that the first section of this book has convinced you that extra weight is bad for you in many, many ways. You should also realize that there are lots of reasons that you and the millions of others like you find yourself in this situation. Now it's time to understand that if you don't commit to this change you will continue to find yourself on a very slippery slope.

REALITY CHECK

Think of the roles that you occupy as a father, son, husband, or brother. Think about your job or your volunteer work, and those who count on you. Realize that you're a very important part of your community. Think how critical you are to your friends for support and encouragement and joy, and to your life partner as a companion and a lover. Consider how your parents need you to look after them and provide company as they age. Think about how your children continue to count on you for strength and advice even when they are fully grown. I want you to start to love yourself and to understand how vitally important you are. In this context, I want you to think about how important it is to all of your connections that you live a long and healthy life. And realize that food abuse is not an indicator of self-love—or, for that matter, of love of your family and friends.

I have a question for every man when he first starts on my program: Before you came to meet me for the first time, how old did you think you'd be when you died?

So how about you? How old do you think you'll be when you die? Before you read any further, take a piece of paper and write this age down, seal it in an envelope, and put it in a drawer where you can refer to it someday. Many men think that they will have the same life span as their father or grandfather or uncles. However, they may have been overweight, abused themselves with food, and shortened their lives.

I'm making you a promise right now: By the time you finish this book, you will have the power to increase your life expectancy, even if you are already 55 or 60 years old. It will take some thinking, some changing, some believing, but I know that you'll have longevity expectations that yesterday might have seemed like a pipe dream.

In my weekly men's presentations I will often ask those who have changed to healthier eating, and have lost 30, 40, 60, or 100 pounds, how many years they now expect to live. Many will say 20 or 30 more years, now that they have reclaimed their lives. They have hope about a future that they once thought they wouldn't see.

I also ask men how many of them have more life insurance on their own life than on their spouse's life. Usually, every single one of the 150 men in the group raises a hand. Men are convinced that they will be the first to go.

What About Our Partners?

Face it; a large insurance policy won't buy your mate companionship, shared future memories, or your love. One time in the Sunday morning group that I run, a very unselfish man came forward and said, "Harvey, that's the very reason I'm doing this for myself; that's the very reason I'm losing my weight. I want to outlive my wife." After a few chuckles from the rest of the guys, he continued, "No, seriously; she's told me many times that in her old age she couldn't stand the thought of suffering alone. I love my wife so much that I plan to do everything in my power to live to over 100 now that I know that I can be healthy and spend my days with the love of my life until she passes away."

This man got applause from the other men after that. You can decide not to be the "designated die-er" if you want. We've been conditioned to believe that thinking about yourself is selfish. But if you put yourself first and get healthy and fit, then you can really take care of those you love.

Wouldn't you agree that it's crazy that you, as a responsible man, perhaps a dad, a husband, brother, or son, would shorten your life or impair your health when you could stop doing that right now? Wouldn't you say you owe yourself a future of health as well as prosperity? Wouldn't you say that the family and community you are a part of should be entitled to have you with them for a long time into the future?

If you are reading this book, you are ready! You want to save your life and live a healthier future. You want to outlive your partner, because you think so much about her or him that you don't want that person to suffer. If you are a caring man, you must be willing to do whatever is necessary to change direction starting now.

Unfortunately, motivation and knowing how to go about it are two decidedly different things. "Many men want to change; few are ready to make changes."

Militancy with yourself is the only thing that can work. The good news is that this section of the book will allow you to focus that militancy on activities that will deliver you results.

MALE PROCRASTINATION

"People procrastinate because they are afraid of the success that they know will result if they move ahead now. Because success carries such a heavy responsibility with it, it is much easier to live on the 'Someday I'll' philosophy."

—Denis Waitley

You need to get into the game if you want to win. What triggered you to read this book? The name? The cover? Did someone buy it for you? You have known for some time, or someone close to you has known, that you have to do something. But what? You didn't realize there was a program and philosophy that would work for you. The guys whose pictures you see in this book were just like you at one time. You too can become a Brooker man. You have the power within you to change, and now I'm going to provide you with a road map that will lead you to the results you need.

Think of this stage as "boot camp." You've got to follow my eating program, and deal with the external saboteurs that can put you off course. You've got to eliminate your own bad influence. In my groups, I call him "Slick," and he's the devil within that tells you that it's alright to order deep fried chicken wings and French fries "because I'm out with the boys." In five years' time, you'll be able to look back and see why you kept the weight off. It is your dedication at the outset of this project that sets the firm foundation on which you can build. So the next 90 days will be vital. Executing what you are reading here will help you accomplish your dreams. The alternative is that you do nothing and pack this book away on a shelf with all the other self-help books that you've never followed. It's your choice. If you read on, I want you to roll up your sleeves and do what we discuss in these pages. I promise that if you do, you'll never look back!

Men Should Make a Project of Learning How to Eat Properly

My idea of a project is a specific plan with a projected outcome. I want you to make it an ongoing project to get and stay healthy. As a man, I learned that losing weight was not just about food. After getting to my ideal weight, I found that it was a philosophy, a way of thinking about others, and of course myself. I wanted to control my health and my state of mind so that I could contribute to the world about me. To do this, and to help you, I had to plan and think of becoming and staying healthy. This could not be a fuzzy "nice to have"; I needed a structure to make it doable. The only difference is that every other project has a completion date. This one is ongoing.

All projects should have two states:

· The current status: where you are right now.
· The completed status: what it will look like when completed.

An architect already knows what the project will look like before the hole for the new building has been dug. In your project—getting to a healthy weight—remember, the way we start projects has a direct affect on the outcome. If we do our best to think out a plan that will account for all the variables that will be thrown our way, then we've greatly increased our odds for success.

Imagine this: You decide to start your own business. You rent an office, put some phone lines in, hire a secretary, lease some furnishings, and hire an assistant, but do not have any idea where you will sell your products or how much you should charge. Of course, you would be doomed to failure. And just as surely as a business project with that kind of approach is doomed to fail, factors like a soft market, heavy competition, and poor staff are blamed. The fact is that your enterprise will have failed because defined goals were not laid out at the preliminary stage of setting up the business venture, and there were no contingency plans set to come into play if the business environment changed.

The same would be true if you were going to renovate the basement and tore down the old walls and supports, and started hammering up the new drywall without any plan. The result would be a disaster.

That is why you have to think of your weight management challenge as a project. If you are reading this book and you suspect that you need to lose 40 pounds and say to yourself, "I think I'll give it a try" but don't make your own plan and only pay attention to half of the advice, it won't work! You must have clearly defined benchmarks and a program that will achieve them.

Write Down Everything You Eat on Your Current Diet

Soon you'll be using my simple and quick Daily Eating Awareness Record that is tailored to my ONE**80** Plan, but it is important to first pull out a regular journal or notepad, and take a few days or a week to record everything you currently eat. And think about your eating style: What do you eat for snacks? Do you sometimes binge? Do you skip meals? Are you a fast eater? Do you fall for junk food on a regular basis? Do you stuff yourself? Do you find yourself eating before you go to bed?

In your notebook, make careful notes of everything, and I mean everything, that you eat and drink over the next week. Do your best to estimate all amounts. A can of Coke. An eight-ounce steak. A handful of peanuts. The estimate will not be perfect, but it will give you an excellent barometer of your present eating habits. Try and note the foods and times of day as soon after eating as possible. (You're much less likely to forget.) Don't worry if it seems to be taking up a lot of time; you'll only be doing this for a week before switching to the Daily Eating Awareness Record, which takes only a few minutes every day. Behave during this week as you always have, all your adult life. Don't eat or drink anything more or less. This sheet or document should be stored for future reference. It will provide an interesting contrast to your future eating behavior.

Write Down Your Thoughts

In that same notebook, write out how you feel physically. Do you have energy at the end of the day? How do you sleep? Can you still do the things that you used to do when you were in college? Do you have any weight-related ailments that you've discussed with your doctor? Make as exhaustive a list as possible.

Now in a second section write down your mental state. How do you feel about yourself? How do others feel about you? Are you confident? Do you feel that you're performing at work as well as you could? How does your mate feel about you? How's your sex life? If you feel that you're in physical or emotional pain, write it down and remember it.

Don't forget, you'll be storing this for future reference. It will become a profound source of motivation as your health begins to improve.

Write Down Your Benchmarks

We won't talk about "goals" here; to me, a goal is an end, as in an end weight. "If I don't lose 30 pounds by Christmas, I'm quitting." This diet mentality sets you up for failure.

The fact is that neither you nor I know the weight that you'll be when you've been eating properly for four years, five years, or 15 years. It doesn't matter, because it will be the right weight for you.

I'm asking you to change your eating behavior for the rest of your life, so think about benchmarks that will determine whether or not you are staying on track. Use your notes from your present to set up a contrasting state that would appeal to you for the rest of your life. Write out benchmarks that would demonstrate that you were doing the things that will keep you on track. They could be as simple as eating a proper breakfast each day of the week. It could be that you've cut out fried foods. Maybe within a certain number of weeks you want to start walking for half an hour a day.

Write Down Your Contingency Plans

This is the moment when you identify the "triggers" that cause you to overeat . . . those moments when "Slick" has the opportunity to creep onto your shoulder and whisper into your ear. Once you recognize your triggers, you can—and must—plan in advance for how to deal with them. Start by examining which people, events, or circumstances make you feel unfocused. Is it long work hours, a cranky boss, a full schedule, or a relationship issue?

Record every trigger you can think of. Then write down what you will do when you encounter those triggers to fend off your usual over-eating response. If these events actually occur, write down when they occurred, your response, and how well it worked.

Yearly Review

Your new life is about going forward, but you need to learn as you go, so plan to have a regular, annual review on your progress. Review your success in terms of your benchmarks that you had for that year, and adjust them for the year that is approaching.

In the coming chapters you're going to learn how to get started. To be sure that the project is going to work, there are a few very important principles that you need to commit to.

Principle 1: Make this a priority in your life.

Excess weight is putting your health and well-being in jeopardy. Where are you going to be 10, 20, or 30 years from now? Have you really, finally decided this is it?

Think about the project every day until you're able to live a healthy life because it has become a natural part of who you are. On a scale of 1 to 10, just how important is this issue of weight loss and a healthier future to you? It should be a 10. Why? Because with good health everything is better; anything is possible; you'll be able to seriously consider doing those things that you always wanted to do. If you want to know how important health is, just ask those who are restricted in dozens of ways. Let them tell you how their plans fall short because of untimely illness, bypass operations, and other similar events.

With good health and a slimmer body, energy for everything increases. At work you can demonstrate more productivity and a sharper mind. For pleasure, you'll have more energy to participate in sports and other leisure activities with your kids and your mate.

Resolve to make this a priority and you will avoid the regrets later on!

Principle 2: Clear the negative thoughts.
Many men who have joined my organization have believed they would live a shortened life. It may be that a member of their family was overweight and died prematurely and they felt that they would suffer the same fate. It might be that life had become less joyful and they didn't care to live a long time. In some ways saying that they didn't care whether they lived long became an excuse to behave however they pleased. After all, if you rationalize that you can't have any effect on the length of your life, then you can easily give yourself permission to eat and drink and smoke as much as you like. This is complete bullshit.

I don't care what belief system you have, or where you believe you'll be in the hereafter. As far as we know we only have one shot at this life, with this group of family, friends, and co-workers. If that's the case, then wouldn't curiosity make you want to make the best of it? Why shouldn't you live to 95 and see what it has to offer?

The other reason that men are negative is because they've tried to get control before and have suffered a number of failures. Well, you haven't failed; you've just gone about your effort in the wrong way. I'm here to tell you that there's a process that works and that has no gimmicks.

Principle 3: Visualize the results that you want.
Sit in a quiet place for a moment and see yourself in a great suit walking down the street, feeling very proud of the way you look. Athletes use visualization to make themselves successful, and I want you to use it as a form of self-actualization.

Ralph Waldo Emerson said, "What the mind of man can conceive, he can believe and achieve."

I think that it's a safe bet to assume that anyone who invents anything, be it a product, a service, or a company, must imagine it before it can become a reality. In Toronto, an architect imagined how the first retractable roof on a stadium would work before the creation of the SkyDome.

Just when you think that people have created everything possible, an individual has the will and the audacity to take an idea to the next logical step. I love this: even before the twentieth century began, the U.S. patent office stated that everything that could be invented had been! Yet there have been more inventions in the last 25 years than there were in the whole prior history of mankind.

Clearly if we can imagine something and become determined to make it happen, then it can become a reality. Sir Edmund Hilary envisioned climbing Mount Everest, and made it a reality.

You must understand that this is true for you as well.

Believe that those who truly love you have the right and expectation for you to be at your very best health and you will see yourself fulfilling your true role as a father, son, husband, brother, or friend.

The next thing that you need to do is imagine how you would like to appear and feel when you hit your ideal body weight. It may be that you'd like to feel like you were in college. Maybe you weren't in such great shape at that time and would like to feel even better than that. The important thing is to take the time to have a very clear visual image. If it's vague, you won't get there. The more clarity and intensity you visualize with, the more this future vision becomes an active part of who you are today. That is the profound power of visualization.

In the past you allowed circumstances to create your state of health and the way you looked. This time, you will dictate your own circumstances and you will create the results you desire.

Principle 4: Believe that you can achieve.

For you to achieve your appropriate weight, you must believe in this project. Teams rarely win if they don't believe in the strategy that their coach has devised.

Why should you believe? Well, first of all, keep reading, and decide for yourself if what I'm writing makes sense to you. Second, have a look at my track record. Look at the pictures of my Brooker men: real people, from all walks of life, who have lost large numbers of pounds and maintained their new weight. You are not at a healthy weight right now because some part of you does not believe that it is possible. But it is.

Roger Bannister ran hundreds of miles and trained endlessly, driven by his belief that he could break the four-minute mile. When he became the first man to run one mile in less than four minutes, others realized that the impossible was possible, and in no time many others had broken the mark, because of his determined belief.

If you believe, as others have, that my strategy makes sense, and that you will succeed, then you'll be willing to put in the extra effort, even when you encounter setbacks. Believe that you will succeed.

Principle 5: Be tenacious.

No one can do everything in life easily. If it were going to be really easy for you to keep the weight off, you wouldn't be in the situation that you're in today.

Learn from role models who were born with an innate understanding of getting things done by being tenacious. Ernest Shackleton led an ill-fated trek to the South Pole in the early 1900s. When his ship was crushed and stranded in the ice, he was determined to get his men out of Antarctica alive. Over months, he led his men through the most appalling conditions to the coast, where he left them sheltered under an overturned row boat. He then took several men and rowed through the ice floes to secure a rescue ship from South America. When he returned to get the men he had left behind, they could not believe that he'd actually made it. Due to his sheer will and determination he was able to overcome the disaster and get everyone out of Antarctica alive.

To use an inspiring personal example, my wife, Helen, who never felt she was good at school, was a high school drop-out when we got married. She realized that absolutely nothing stood between her and her education other than a lot of effort, and she not only finished high school; she got a law degree in her late forties.

For you to accomplish losing weight and maintaining your weight loss, you're going to need to dig down into your resources and demonstrate that you have real tenacity. You may not think that it's in you, but all of us have demonstrated it. If we only did the things in life that came easily, and never tried the things that were difficult, I believe that we would be bored to tears. Life would be pretty meaningless.

Think of something that you tried that at first felt impossible. It could have been learning to ski as an adult. It might be that you moved to a different country where you discovered that you actually could learn a new language. Maybe you took up a difficult instrument, or made close friends with someone who you initially found difficult. There's no question that the greatest satisfaction comes from those achievements where you really had to demonstrate a personal ability to stick to the task, even when no one else believed you could succeed.

Successful people are often described as "lucky" or having "what it takes," and maybe some have a bit of that. But most successful people are those who apply the rule of 50 percent inspiration and 50 percent dedication. Those two states of mind give them what they need to "make it." You'll need them, too: tenacity and ambition.

Principle 6: Always be prepared.

Just like the Boy Scouts, we must be prepared. Your future is that of "a chronic restrained eater."

In the next chapter, I'll provide you with the practical tips to help you through the typical situations that derail weight loss. But to be successful you need to be prepared for the moments when hypoglycemia (low blood sugar) sets in. A prime example is that time around four o'clock in the afternoon. If you haven't planned for it, hunger strikes, insanity sets in, and you fall off the health cart directly onto a muffin and coffee. If you do this, it will cause you to pick on yourself: "I'm failing again." I'm no good at this." First, remember that *no one can be reasonable when hunger dominates his thoughts*. Second, all of this can be avoided by being prepared.

You have to think ahead about what you're going to eat if you're traveling on an airplane, or if you're invited to someone's home for dinner. What food will you purchase for your own house? Don't get caught with your plans down. Think your way through to the next eating situation. Avoid and abstain from unhealthy eating by planning and preparing!

Principle 7: Patience is a virtue.

Don't be disappointed with slower losses, and don't get too high because of quick ones. Just lean back, relax, stay focused, and give yourself time to learn and to change. It's a principle that will guide you to assured results.

In this and in any other success you want in life, patience is mandatory. In this time of instant everything—instant soups, instant communications, instant dinners, and instant millionaires—we can get fooled into believing only in fast and faster. You may know some people who've lost weight quickly, but for most it will take some time. After all, it took some time to put on the weight.

If you happen to be someone who loses more slowly, so what? Each day that passes, no matter what the weight loss, is a day closer to your personal goal. And with each day of dedication to this project, you have another day of knowing that you are on the right track, the only track to solving this dilemma.

Principle 8: Pursue this with a passion!

This has to become not just a belief, but a knowing so deep inside you that it's a fire that says: Yes, I can!

Look, in the end, it doesn't matter if problems are the cause of your weight gain or weight gain is the cause of your problems. Passionate people get the job done.

They believe passionately that they are the masters of their own destiny. They never give up and never give in, and if they rest for a moment they soon wake to their calling again. They always remember why they are doing this.

They never forget the pain and the fear that brought them to this commitment, and they are going to do business—the business of living life as never before!

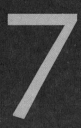

MY COMMON SENSE RULES FOR MEN'S WEIGHT LOSS

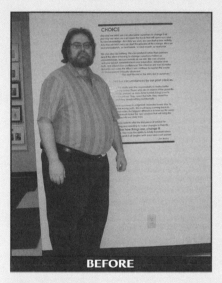

BEFORE

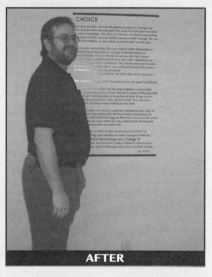

AFTER

If you'd asked me in February last year if I was successful, I'd have answered, "Of course." I was quite successful in my career and as a parent, self-confident, happy, well off financially, and living the good life.

I now know that I was also successful at being a fat man. I had accepted the need for some accessories—CPAP machine to overcome sleep apnea, cholesterol and blood pressure medications, and a glucose level tester that was starting to complain to me. I had the coping strategies for being fat—I'd long since buried any desire to look good; I'd accepted the need for "seatbelt extenders" on airplanes, and I had the defensive humor all lined up to help me overcome the stigma of being fat. (My best talent? Ballast. My tailor's name? Omar the Tentmaker.)

Sadly, I'd even accepted the pains that are related to being fat—sore hips, breathlessness, sleeping with an air pump. I was unable to get life insurance, and I fully expected to have a heart attack by the time I was 60. . . and had accepted it. As a fat man, I had successfully learned to bury my pride, stop caring about looks or insults, and ignore the fact that I was killing myself.

Then along came Harvey Brooker to change all that. Thanks to his program, I'm feeling good. I have the energy to enjoy life again. I'm getting involved in the community for the first time in many years. At 54 years old, I'm just starting to enjoy splurging on new clothes and paying attention to my looks.

I no longer avoid that extra trip upstairs, because I can do several trips without being out of breath. I've ridden my bicycle 900 kilometers this past summer, and have come to cherish the time that I have out exercising, listening to music, and relaxing (in a healthy way!). I have much more energy and am up at 6:00 a.m. daily, ready to go. I'm losing the pains associated with morbid obesity as I shed the pounds, and I'm losing the old attitude and coping strategies (tragedies!) at the same time.

Nine months (and 60 pounds) later, I'm just now achieving true success. Instead of being successfully fat, I'm successful at being healthier, more energetic, more motivated, and more positive. Thanks to Harvey Brooker, I'm just getting started on "ME, version 2.0," with lots more to come!

John R. Snyder

There's something about trying to lose weight that causes people to lose their sanity. Over years and years of successfully working with men, I've proven to myself and my clients that common sense is quite uncommon in this industry, and so I'm going to share the guiding principles that you can start to apply as part of your commitment to my ONE**80** Plan. Photocopy this list and revisit it as often as you need to:

THE ONE80 COMMON SENSE RULES

1. Eat food, not food products
2. Develop your own hunger gauge
3. Keep your hunger below 6
4. Weigh yourself regularly
5. Weigh your food
6. Eat slowly
7. Drink water
8. Try one new food every week
9. Avoid coffee and tea
10. Cut back on alcohol
11. Don't skip meals
12. Don't eat bread after lunch
13. Eat healthy snacks, especially in the afternoon
14. Eat your protein last
15. Reverse meals on occasion
16. Don't fry your food
17. Pay attention while you eat
18. Stay away from "mystery" foods
19. Eliminate temptation
20. Choose a support partner
21. Equip your kitchen
22. Learn the rules of food shopping
23. Stick to the plan always

1. EAT FOOD, NOT FOOD PRODUCTS

Not so long ago, all food was nutritious. Unfortunately, that is no longer the case. As we've discussed, the food industry is now producing a great deal of prepared and packaged products (I don't want to call it food) that you and your body don't need. This book will teach you how to avoid these temptations, and show you what it is that you really do need.

The same is true of supplements. You'll never have a sustainable weight loss program if you need to forever-after buy special products or supplements in order to keep the weight off. You have already decided not to waste money on "magic" diet pills, herbs, or whatever else comes momentarily into fashion. It's common sense to me that any program that's going to have a chance of success must be based on real food, and that food must be available right at your corner grocer, any time you want!

I've learned how to make sure I'm always satisfied and full, without consuming unnecessary calories, and without taking supplements, and I'll show you how, too.

2. DEVELOP YOUR OWN HUNGER GAUGE

This concept has helped the men in my classes tremendously, and yet it's something that few of us who are not in the business ever think about. Take a moment and analyze how you feel when you have eaten a good meal and are completely satisfied. This sensation gives you a hunger gauge of 0. Now imagine what it's like if you've missed a meal and are starving. Your hunger gauge in this instance will be 10. The trick is to pay attention to how you are feeling at all times and never let your hunger gauge slip past 5.5. This will keep you from getting so hungry that you binge (eating anything and everything, nonstop) on food that you don't really need.

3. KEEP YOUR HUNGER BELOW 6

So many men make the mistake of starving themselves in an attempt to manage their weight, and then when they finally allow themselves to eat, they binge. Does this sound familiar to you? It may seem counterintuitive, but in order to lose weight effectively, you need to fill up with nutritious low-fat foods and never starve yourself. If you eat three nutritious meals a day and snack sensibly, you will never arrive home from work or from a long drive starving. Carry snacks with you and keep your eye on your hunger gauge.

When you've made it through the day, make sure that you never go to bed hungry. It is best to not eat late at night, but if you've been in the habit of eating too much, there's a risk that you'll wake up and raid the refrigerator. Eventually you won't need to eat in the late evenings, but if you do at first, make a light healthy snack to help settle you down. I recommend a half a cup of unsweetened apple sauce with 3/4 of a cup of plain no fat yogurt with a teaspoon of diet jam added for flavor. This will have you sleeping like a baby all night long.

Most men do just fine with the no-hunger rule until they are invited out and realize that they can't control themselves when the food arrives. Whether you are invited to a friend's house for a meal or you're at a business dinner or a banquet, eat a small meal in advance to curb your hunger.

4. WEIGH YOURSELF REGULARLY, ON THE SAME SCALE, AT THE SAME TIME OF THE WEEK

Clearly, to gauge your progress, you must weigh yourself regularly. I know that like all men who are into instant gratification, you're going to want to see how you are doing every day. This is not the way to succeed! Instead, you should choose a day and a time each week, and stick to it. Weigh yourself on the same scale at the same time of day on the same day each week.

Don't be tempted to weigh yourself any more often than that. If you do, you can be faced with two unfortunate results. First, if you get an overly positive weight loss, you can be tempted to slack off your efforts because you think that you've achieved your goal for the week. This can cause you to slip back. Or, if you're not losing the weight that you'd hoped, you can become discouraged, and this may cause you to give up prematurely—nothing seems to be working. Because your weight fluctuates naturally during the day, choosing the same time will ensure the most accurate measurement of how you are doing over the long run.

5. WEIGH YOUR FOOD AS WELL AS YOURSELF—IT'S GOING TO BE PART OF YOU

Okay, you're going to have to get involved in the kitchen if you're going to be successful! This is because, until you can accurately ballpark the proper proportion size, it's necessary to measure all cooked foods with a scale (measuring in ounces). Not only is it important to weigh the food after it is cooked, but you should also make sure, if it's protein, that you weigh only the edible part after the bone and the skin have been removed. This makes it possible for you to truly control your portions.

Previously, your idea of a serving of protein meant a steak that was half the size of your dinner plate. If you want steak, you should be eating about a five-ounce portion—about the size of a deck of cards. In essence, you're going to be learning to practice chronic restrained eating, which is not a concept that most men have ever thought about. If the M-word worries you, I can tell you from experience that moderation is better than outright denial. You may be wondering how you're going to be able to pass on your favorite foods in order to lose weight. Do you love barbecued chicken? Just keep the portion to five ounces. Once you get familiar with the recommended portion sizes, you will find the portions on my ONE**80** Plan easy and satisfying, whether you're making your own on the grill or eating out.

6. EAT YOUR MEALS SLOWLY

Do you race through your meal as if it were some sort of athletic contest? This is a very bad habit, because it takes your body some time to signal to your brain that it's had enough to eat. In fact, research says that it takes at least 20 minutes for your body to register that it's full. You may still feel hungry even though your stomach is full. This is one of the problems with fast food, even sandwiches—you can gulp all of it down in less than 10 minutes.

It's easy to get around this. First, get in the habit of starting your meals with a large salad or a bowl of vegetable soup. This will both extend the length of the meal, and also make sure that you are getting lots of nutrient-rich foods throughout the day. Also, always sit down for meals, and make it a habit to use a knife and fork, even at lunch. If you brown-bag lunch, try not to eat sandwiches. Sandwiches tend to be eaten so quickly you hardly get a chance to chew them, and we just don't seem to get the full feeling that is so necessary for most men.

You can also choose foods that take longer to eat (think of the time it takes to eat a chicken breast with rice and vegetables, compared to two slices of pizza); that's another way of allowing your brain the opportunity to catch up with your body.

7. WATER YOURSELF REGULARLY

It's a silly heading, but it's good advice. Every part of the body, from cognitive function to digestion, needs adequate water to ensure proper functioning. The general rule is to have eight glasses of water per day, plus another one for every 25 pounds of weight that you need to lose. If you can't stomach that much plain water, then jazz it up with some fresh-sliced lemon or lime. Water fills you up with no calories, and it flushes out toxins. Did you know that thirst can mimic hunger? Often when you think that you are hungry, you are actually thirsty. Try drinking a glass of water and waiting half an hour before having that snack, and you might discover that you don't need the food anymore.

8. TRY ONE NEW FOOD PER WEEK

Men are notorious for getting stuck in an eating pattern. This is your chance to break out! Most of us get into an eating rut, and if you're overweight, chances are that the rut contains many foods that are high in calories and low in nutrition. Make an action list and try some different foods every week. It doesn't matter whether it is a kind of fish you haven't had before, or a new vegetable, like purple carrots or yellow tomatoes: learn about the wide variety of tastes that can help to make your new menu interesting and exciting.

Become familiar with the fruits and vegetables sections of your local supermarket. There are dozens of items that you may discover for the very first time. There are about 12 types of lettuces; try romaine, Bibb, iceberg, and radicchio. Carrots come washed and peeled for a great afternoon sugar pick-me-up or to go in your salads. There are English and regular cucumbers. Try Belgian endive and four or five sweet peppers in different colors. Remember, in food selection we eat by taste and by sight. So if something is appealing to the eye, it will increase your culinary interest. Fruit is also in the same category. Look for new fruits to try; you will find it is worthwhile.

9. AVOID COFFEE AND TEA

We are inclined to use coffee or tea for a lift during the day. Unfortunately, both coffee and tea stimulate your liver to pump sugar into your bloodstream. While this may sound like a good way to get energy, a sugar high is always followed by a sugar low, and sugar lows can make us feel ferociously hungry. A healthy drink alternative could include herbal teas, plain water, or carbonated water (that doesn't have any salt). Breaking the coffee habit may seem difficult at first, but the long-term weight loss will make the effort worthwhile.

10. CUT BACK ON ALCOHOL

If you are adding alcohol as part of your program for that day, consider ordering a spritzer of wine instead of a glass of wine. If you are just beginning the ONE80 Plan, I suggest that you abstain from having any alcohol; it stimulates your appetite and makes it harder to maintain self-control.

11. DON'T SKIP MEALS, ESPECIALLY BREAKFAST

Many men avoid what I consider to be the most important meal: breakfast. A full third of my male clients do not eat breakfast at all. Many others claim to have breakfast, but I discover, after consulting with them, that their breakfast typically consists of too little (a glass of citrus juice and a coffee), or too much (mountains of bacon and fried eggs).

Breakfast is an essential meal, the spark that lights your metabolism and gives you the energy to start your day. Beginning your day with a healthy meal ensures that your blood sugar levels do not drop too low, causing a surge of hunger and cravings. These cravings cause the classic mid-morning "muffin and coffee break" that so many are accustomed to. High-fat, high-calorie foods like donuts, croissants, bagels or muffins not only cause us to gain weight themselves, they actually make us hungrier—the perfect set-up for that huge lunch or four-course dinner. Did you know that a single muffin can contain up to 500 calories, most of them from fat? Not to mention the sugar content! By having a balanced, healthy breakfast each day, perhaps a couple of poached eggs on multigrain toast, or hot cereal with fruit (no fried bacon and eggs, please), you will actually consume fewer calories throughout the day.

12. DON'T EAT BREAD AFTER LUNCH

While whole wheat bread provides good nutrition and can certainly be a part of your program, bread is often eaten as a comfort food. Also, all breads are not created equal. Those French sticks that come in the bread basket prior to many meals are laden with calories that you just don't need, particularly as you are following that snack with a real meal. If you are sticking to the rules above, you'll be starting your meal with a salad now, so that one will be easy to avoid. I try and avoid bread after lunch. You'll find that it's a great habit for you as well.

13. STOP THE MID-AFTERNOON SLUMP

In the mid-afternoon many people experience crash time. That is when the blood sugar levels seem to drop suddenly. You know the feeling: it's four o'clock and the office snack bar and vending machines are all calling your name. "We've got potato chips, we've got chocolate bars, and we're only a few steps away." You need to be prepared. Keep a bag of mini carrots on hand. Pull an apple, orange, banana, or pear out of your drawer. Any of these alternatives can create a quick afternoon pick-me-up, without fat and extra calories. Instead of succumbing to disaster, you'll be filling up with healthy foods and getting lots of vitamins and fiber at the same time.

14. EAT YOUR PROTEIN LAST AT DINNER

As we've said before, men are protein eaters! Dinner has traditionally been the largest meal of the day in North America, and nearly all the men I've met start by eating their protein. In fact, many men will have second helpings of meat before they've touched any of their vegetables (if they eat them at all). This means that they are not getting the other nutrients that they need to be healthy. Here's an easy way to reduce that fat intake. Start your meal with two or three vegetables. As you refill your vegetable portion, begin eating your protein. This helps you eat your proteins slowly at dinner, and allows your stomach time to signal that it is full. Because you will be having smaller protein portions than you are used to now, this will make the transition surprisingly easy—you'll find you are satisfied with less, and your energy levels will dramatically increase.

15. REVERSE MEALS OCCASIONALLY

There will be times when you're out for lunch and faced with a situation where you are hungry and there are some good healthy choices on the menu. Occasionally it's okay to have your dinner as your noon meal. This can be particularly appropriate when others are eating a larger meal and you don't want to be just sitting there eating a much smaller meal. It can provide a nice change of pace, as long as you remember to have your lunch at dinner time. In other words you are completely reversing your meals and dinner will be lighter.

16. DON'T BE A FRY GUY

Chances are that for some time, you've been living on a diet of fat-soaked goodies. One of the ways that you can get control of your weight is to learn to eat the same food and simply broil, boil, roast, steam, or bake your meals. Liven the meals up by adding lemon juice and herbs. Remove all visible fat from meats before cooking. Healthy meals don't need to be bland, and there are lots of healthy recipes at the end of the book that taste great and will keep you on track. Remember, nothing tastes as good as thin feels.

17. PAY ATTENTION TO WHAT YOU ARE EATING

How many times have you been watching TV and munching away on some potato chips, blissfully unaware of how many you've had until you've reached the bottom of the bag? Some people like to snack while they are on the computer, or while they are driving. You've got to slow down, stop, and pay attention to what you are putting in your mouth. Do your eating at the dinner table, and plan for snack food that is low in calories and high in nutrition.

18. STAY AWAY FROM "MYSTERY" FOODS

You may know the name of the recipe, but if you didn't make it yourself, then it is a "mystery food." Chilies, beef barley soup, lasagna—they all taste wonderful, but it's impossible to tell how many calories you are consuming or what they have been made with. The best advice that I can provide is that unless you are making them yourself, these kinds of foods should be avoided.

19. ELIMINATE TEMPTATION

Make your home a safe haven! The old adage "out of sight, out of mind" works here. Don't play games with yourself: clean out your pantry and refrigerator, and get rid of all the high-fat, high-sugar goodies that can tempt you. I know how easy it is to hide food, but in a weak moment you know where to find it. Your home should be your one totally safe place in the world. It needs to be free from temptation and anxiety. Who needs to face the stress of resisting the wrong foods in your own home? Talk to your family, your roommate, your spouse. Tell them how important this project is to you, and them.

Sometimes clients of mine have used their kids as an excuse for having junk food in the house. Childhood obesity is also a problem in our culture! Don't buy junk food for your kids. You may think that you're simply giving them a treat, but a treat soon becomes a routine part of their behavior and in the long run, you are not doing them a favor. Don't fall for the trap that your denial of treats for them is not fair. Having that junk food in the house is an unfair temptation for you when you are starting out and it sets patterns for them that can eventually lead to childhood obesity. Teach your family and children how to have healthy eating behaviors and how to make the right choices.

20. CHOOSE A SUPPORT PARTNER

Clearly the first and most important support for your project is you. Think of times you've succeeded and remember the determination you had then. This is the effort you'll have to bring to this program.

Enlisting family support is also important. After all, your health is important to them, and you're with them every day. You must explain the importance of the program to them and they must also agree to be tough with you. This positive reinforcement will be critical to your success.

Looking for a personal trainer who works in your vicinity is another great option. Interview several in order to make sure that you get the right one. The individual that you choose must be willing to work to understand the program and your goals and to hold your feet to the fire. The benefit of personal trainers is that they can ease you back into exercise as you start to reduce your weight to its normal level.

You can also go to our website, www.itsdifferentformen.com. This link contains our program and will allow you to network with other men who are in the same situation as you. This group support can be invaluable in keeping you on track.

21. EQUIP YOUR KITCHEN

Everything listed below is cheap, easy to find, and incredibly helpful.

- **Food scale:** You will need an ounce scale to weigh your foods daily. It is very important to learn how to measure your food for accuracy; it will give you a good idea, in particular, of just what a five-ounce portion of protein looks like. The discipline of weighing your food daily will make it easier for you to eat similar portions when you are outside your home. Eventually, you'll be able to size food in your mind, but not when you start.

- **Steamer and wok:** You will also need a steamer to cook fast and tasty fish, vegetables, and rice, and a wok to prepare vegetables and low-fat stir-fries. It's not an accident that people from Asia who cook with these tools instead of frying pans and casserole dishes suffer a lower rate of weight issues than their North American counterparts.

- **Grill:** A useful North American invention for fast grilling of chicken and fish is the George Foreman grill. That or something like it can become a valuable ally in eating properly.

- **Blender:** If you don't have one already, get a blender to make delicious low-calorie shakes.

- **Recipe books:** Cookbooks are also an important tool in your project. Keep your meals interesting and varied. Go to your local bookstore or get on the web and browse through the cookbook section. Look for easy, low-calorie recipes for chicken, fish, vegetables, and soups. There are cookbooks with recipes for low-cal desserts. You will be surprised to discover a whole world of wonderful and delicious foods that are low in fat and sugar. You'll find balanced, healthy recipes at the end of the book to get you started. If you don't cook, ask your spouse, your mother, or your roommate to try one or two of the recipes. If you go about this with the right attitude, it can be fun.

That covers you pretty well on the equipment side. On the ingredient side, as well as everything you are going to read about in the next chapter, it's very important to have a well-equipped spice rack to enhance the flavor of the food. It is worth the minimal cost and effort, so add some zest to your program. With a little bit of effort, your meals will be varied and delicious!

22. LEARN THE RULES OF FOOD SHOPPING

- **...with a list**   Rule number one is to shop with a list. This helps you avoid the spontaneous purchase of something that you shouldn't have. Creating a list means that you'll be thinking about what you're going to eat in the coming week, which will also help to avoid the drive-thru meals that are so appealing when the fridge is empty! Make sure that you're thinking about what you'd like to have for snacks and buy those at the grocery store so you are not caught without them.

- **...when you're not hungry**   Never go to the supermarket hungry. Have you ever noticed that everything looks fantastic when you're hungry? Wandering those food-filled aisles then makes it way too easy to impulse shop, especially those grab-and-go packaged foods filled with salt and sugar and fat. If you know that you're going to be shopping when you are out and about, bring along a light snack to eat about 10 minutes before you know you're going to be in the store. With a full belly, it's much easier to resist the chips, candy, and other bad food choices that will surround you.

- **...on the outside perimeter of the store**   The outside perimeter of the store is where the whole foods are kept: fruit, vegetables, whole grains, and low-fat dairy products. In the middle aisles you will find the processed products—the ones most likely to contain excess sugar, salt, and preservatives.

- **...while reading the labels**   In order to make good food choices, you must discipline yourself to read labels. There is a lot of information there! Of course, you will probably want to pay close attention to the fat contents of products. Let's say that a one-ounce serving of hard cheese has a total of 80 calories with seven grams of fat. To figure out the percentage of fat in the cheese, simply multiply the fat grams by nine and divide that result by the total number of calories. Seven grams of fat times nine equals 63 calories. And 63 divided by 80 equals 78 percent of fat in that hard cheese! This is a product you will probably choose to pass by when shopping for lower-fat items to bring home.

Also, watch the wording on labels. For example, "wheat flour" does not mean whole-wheat flour. The best rule to follow is the less processed the item, the better. Be careful of products labeled "light." This does not necessarily mean "low-calorie"—it could mean light in color (light olive oil). Read the labels on margarine, crackers, and breads, and stay away from products that have hydrogenated oil. Hydrogenated oils turn into trans fats. Remember how bad that kind of fat is for your body. Don't buy anything that contains palm or coconut oil. Don't be fooled by so-called "low-fat" products. Very often the fat is replaced by increased levels of sugar, which will convert into fat in your body anyway: you'll be no further ahead with that low-fat alternative.

- **. . .by choosing healthy alternatives** It's important that you find healthy substitutes for the foods that you won't be indulging in anymore. Long-term weight loss is only possible if you change the way that you are eating today by replacing old habits with new ones.

The good news is that most of your old unhealthy choices can easily be replaced with great foods that will help get you to your goal. Don't buy frozen french fries; buy a baking potato and get a lemon or some salsa to liven it up. In this simple example, you avoid taking in fat and empty calories and gain important fiber and vitamins.

Given the immense variety of foods available to us, it's simple to replace unhealthy selections with nutritious alternatives. Soya-based products have come a long way. Try one of the meatless burgers or wiener substitutes; it's very hard to tell that you're not eating the real thing. Want an omelet, and need to avoid the high-cholesterol egg yolks? Simplify your cooking by buying only the egg whites. You can usually find packages of these in the refrigerated dairy section of your supermarket. If you don't want that extra expense, discard two yolks when you're making a three-egg omelet—you'll hardly notice the difference.

Eating healthy doesn't mean avoiding meat entirely. Just increase the number of times that you make healthier choices, such as skinless chicken and fish, instead of beef or lamb, which are filled with heart-clogging saturated fat.

23. CHANGE HOW YOU EAT OUTSIDE THE HOME

• **Restaurants**   A restaurant is simply a retail store that carries a certain line and is trying to get and keep your business. As a result, there is no need for you to be intimidated or feel limited to order exactly what appears on the menu. You have the right to ask for foods to be prepared in a way that is healthy for you. All restaurants cater to issues around allergies. It is perfectly legitimate to ask them to cater to your choices around your health. A smart business owner may not have exactly what you're requesting but should be able to suggest other low-fat alternatives that can be prepared.

It is very important to choose your foods wisely, and also to make sure they are cooked in a healthy way. Fish and chicken should always be grilled, broiled, or roasted without any fat. Ask for your vegetables to be steamed without any butter or oil. Make sure that you tell the server to bring your salad dressing on the side and ask if there is any low-calorie dressing available. Ask for balsamic vinegar or lemon and then put these ingredients on the salad yourself. If you do have salad dressing on the side, dip your fork into the dressing and then put it on the salad so that you can have a taste of the dressing. Usually that is all you will need. If you want dessert, ask them for a bowl of fruit, even if it is not on the menu.

If the portion size on the menu is too large or is not indicated, ask for the amount that you want rather than leaving it up to the restaurant. Most restaurants have scales.

Restaurants are just like any other retail outlets. They want repeat business, so be specific and ask that your food be prepared the way that you want it.

Stay away from buffets and salad bars (or, as I call them, "eating troughs"). I'll often ask my guys, "What did you have for lunch?" The answer is practically always innocent: "Just some salad!"

I ask what kind of salad. "Oh, potato salad with macaroni and mayo." Or "a Waldorf salad." You get the picture; they might as well have had a burger and fries.

It is hard to control how much you eat and what you eat. Most of us want to get our money's worth at a buffet, so we figure we'll eat everything! Select your restaurant carefully. Stay away from places that only serve pizza and wings, or fish and chips restaurants. You may start out with good intentions but it is hard to say no when everything smells good.

Greek restaurants are safe places. Order grilled fish or chicken souvlaki with a side of steamed rice and vegetables.

Most Italian restaurants have fish and chicken on the menu. Order one half cup of pasta as a side order with some steamed vegetables.

Chinese restaurants can be tricky. I would suggest that you stay away from them when you first start your program. When you know the program better and you go to a Chinese restaurant, don't go to a buffet; order from the menu. Steamed fish or lobster is a good idea. Steamed vegetables and rice are great. Ask for your food to be prepared without cornstarch and very light on the oil. Stay away from dishes that are fried or prepared with a sauce of any kind. Those dishes are high in sugar and starch.

- **Fast Food Restaurants**   Fast food restaurants can be a challenge. Many of us have young families and we find ourselves eating in these restaurants, sometimes on a weekly basis. Go to a place that offers salads or grilled chicken burgers—not just a pizza joint. Restaurants that specialize in subs often offer a good choice. Order a turkey sub on whole wheat bread with mustard, lots of veggies, and no mayo. Many fast food places now have a wider variety of healthy foods on their menus.

However, if you know that healthy option is not going to interest you at all, here's the golden rule with fast food restaurants: "Don't go if you can't say no." Just as an alcoholic must avoid going into a bar, you may have to plan to avoid your old fast food haunts. Trying to substitute another food on the menu for your favorite food might not work for you. If you have friends that you used to share your old eating habits with and they want you to continue to eat like them, then you may need to avoid them at mealtimes as well.

Celebrations and Social Events

First, let's talk about parties and weddings or other social gatherings. If you are attending a catered affair, call ahead to where it's being held and tell the caterer that you would prefer to have grilled chicken or fish without any oil and a baked potato with steamed vegetables. Give the person your name so that the server at the affair will be able to serve you the proper meal. You can also call ahead if you are going to a party at a friend's home and ask your host or hostess what they are planning on serving and if you can bring something. If you don't want to call your host or hostess, eat a mini meal like a salad, soup, and couple of pieces of melba toast before you go.

Religious holidays, birthdays, and anniversaries are certainly important events in our lives. These special occasions are always celebrated with good friends and family, almost always with a lot of food and drink. Remember that for right now you need to focus on yourself. Ask your family and friends to make allowances for you and tell them that you just don't eat like you used to. So when the desserts, cakes, and drinks are going around, think about how much better you look and feel. Say, "No, thanks—I don't have to celebrate with a cake. I'm working on this project to make myself healthy and I'll enjoy myself immensely just by being with you."

- **Business Lunches and Seminars** Business meetings and seminars may be important aspects of your career, and they often include snacks, lunches, and dinner. Or, if the meetings are extended over several days, you could be faced with a situation where all of your meals are pre-planned. First bring several fruits with you for coffee breaks. This will stop you from eating muffins or cakes during break time. For the meals themselves, call the hotel or restaurant at which the meeting is being held and speak to the catering manager and pre-order your meals. Be precise about what you want. I am sure that you will find that most restaurants and hotels will be very accommodating. If you are staying at a hotel overnight during a seminar or business meeting, always bring fruit up to your room in the evening. It is important to have something to eat in you room that is satisfying and low in fat and calories.
- **Airplanes** Another tricky situation can be ordering meals in airplanes. If you travel for business, tell your travel agent to have a standing order on your file to always order "low-calorie or low-fat meals" whenever you fly. If the airport allows, it is also a good idea to bring fruit with you on the plane; if you don't eat it then, keep it in your hotel room for a snack.
- **Vacations** You're probably thinking, How can I possibly lose weight when I am on vacation? I always gain at least five pounds! Well, vacationing is relaxing and enjoyable but it is not a time to let all the hard work and weight loss go to waste. You will also enjoy your vacation more if you are feeling good about yourself, your choices, and your health—and the only way to do that is to stay with the program.

Think about where you want to go. It is best not to vacation at an all-inclusive resort or go on a cruise, especially during the first part of your weight loss project. Plan to stay at hotels or resorts where you can either make your breakfast and lunch in your room or order the foods that you require. When eating out, the same good sensible eating or pre-planning applies. If you travel by car for either business trips or vacations, bring along a cooler and stock it with fruit, vegetables, bottled water, juices, and meals, if necessary.

So those are the principles that I've developed that provide the context for managing my ONE**80** Plan. You're now ready to learn the details. It's simple, easy to follow, and guaranteed to work for you, because it never leaves you hungry. I think it's time for you to join the other men whose pictures you've seen throughout the pages of this book. Let's get to it!

MY ONE80 PLAN FOR SUCCESS

8

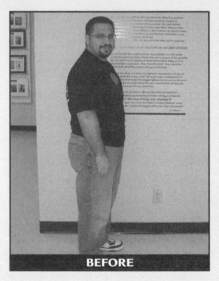

BEFORE

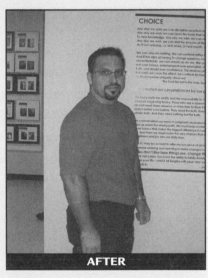

AFTER

My name is Fil. I joined Harvey's program just over a year ago, and have lost between 30 and 35 pounds (from about 245 pounds down to between 210 and 215 pounds) and four inches off my waist (a snug size 40 down to a comfortable size 36). I'm now 41 years old, in good health, eating well; I'm enjoying a lot more of my time, and the activities I can do to fill that time. I've always been a heavy person, with a big and solid frame for my height and age, even as a kid. My slide in lifestyle and weight gain, however, began when I started working full time. Since then, it's been a constant roller coaster of diets, gimmicks, and things that forced me to conform to a plan or program that wasn't realistic. They didn't deal with real food, real life situations, real issues surrounding why we do the things we do with food.

Harvey's program teaches you, nurtures you, supports you, and watches you grow... not in size, but in stature, in knowledge, in self-reliance, in self-conviction, and self-confidence. It empowers you to do it for yourself! And it gives you the tools to make the program your own. Harvey's program does that for all the men that join and stick with it; they lose weight, but gain years—years with family and friends, years for a second career, years they never would have had.

I'm always thinking of food now, but in a good way. I plan in my mind what I'm going to eat today, when am I going to eat it, where am I going, what will they be serving... how do I plan for that event. This is a frame of mind, something that is taught to you, and becomes part of your thought process through the program. I made some changes in how I ate. I started boxing, for a little over an hour, several times a week. I enjoy mountain bike riding a lot more with my son, and downhill skiing with friends.

I can't say enough about the program. I honestly kept it quiet for a while—I wanted to try it; I wanted to see how I did; I wasn't sure. But then I started to tell anyone who asked, because people would see the changes, and want in on it. They wanted "the secret," the "quick fix" (there isn't one) on how I did it. Until you're ready, you won't succeed, but if you're ready, Harvey's program is truly the best and the simplest thing to follow that I've tried. And, I would also add, the last program I will be on.

Fil Magnoli

I invented my ONE**80** Plan to help men make a 180-degree change in their lives—to move away from obesity and sickness and take a new direction towards a long life of health, happiness, and success. This program has been used by my clients over the last 22 years to lose tens of thousands of pounds.

There are three keys to the ONE**80** Plan. The first key is nutrition— you'll be eating for optimum health. The second is portability—the program travels well, because you can find the foods I recommend at any grocery store and at most restaurants, including almost all fast food outlets. The last one is especially important to men: satiety. That means you'll never be hungry, as long as you follow the plan as directed.

The ONE**80** Plan is also incredibly easy to follow. It's so straightforward that you have no choice but success. We're going to cover the nutrition basics so that you have a general understanding of why the program is put together as it is, and then I'll walk you through it. You'll learn to plan your own healthy meals and snacks, and you'll get lots of meal ideas. I'll cover what you can and can't eat, when to eat, and how much to eat. I'm also going to discuss how alcohol fits into this program, and give you some easy strategies for staying on track.

But before we get into the nuts and bolts of the plan, we need to address a very important point: how much weight you need or intend to lose.

WHAT SHOULD YOU WEIGH? THAT'S NATURE'S BUSINESS

Many men who walk through my door ask me what I think their ideal weight should be. I have a simple answer: "That's not my business; it's nature's business!" When I say this, I mean that when you learn how to eat properly and become more active, your weight will naturally level off at a number that is appropriate for you. It makes sense: if you take in fewer calories and burn off more, you will start losing weight. Your ideal weight will not be your choice; you will arrive there by adhering to the principles of the ONE**80** Plan.

When I first interview men and analyze what they are eating, I inevitably find that their calorie intake breaks down about like this: 40 percent from proteins, 40 percent from fats (in the form of meats, hard cheese, dressings, fried foods, and desserts), and 20 percent from carbohydrates. In the case of the carbohydrates, that number is usually laden with simple carbohydrates—white flour, white bread, and white (refined) sugar.

As you would expect with my ONE**80** Plan, I turn the proportions completely around so that they are 55 percent carbohydrates, 30 percent low-fat protein, and 15 percent fat. This allows you to eat fewer calories and attain your "natural weight" while still remaining full.

Here's how it works. It takes approximately 12 calories to maintain each pound of weight that you carry for a day without exercise. Let's say you weigh 250 pounds. 250 x 12 = 3,000 calories. So, at 3,000 calories you would not gain or lose one pound.

It takes 3,500 calories to lose one pound, or to gain one pound. Our ONE**80** plan will give you approximately 2,000 calories per day. The food choices you make will keep you full even though you have cut down dramatically in your calorie intake. So, by cutting down to 2,000 calories per day from the 3,000 that you were previously eating, you will take in 1,000 fewer calories per day. Over the course of a week you will have lost 7,000 calories. This will equal a two-pound weight loss.

Now, let's take you through the math for 220 pounds. 220 x 12 = 2,400 calories. At 2,400 calories you would not gain or lose one pound. But since you are taking in 2,000 calories (or less) per day, you will be taking in approximately 400 fewer calories per day or 2,800 calories per week. So, this will give you a slower loss simply because you don't have as much weight to lose.

At a certain point, your daily calorie intake and your daily calorie needs will level off. That is your real goal weight. That's what I mean by "it's nature's business."

Remember this, however, as you think about what you need to lose: all weight loss improves your life. Any weight loss is an achievement and can provide health benefits. If you are overweight, losing as little as five to 10 percent of your total body weight can improve your health, ability to function, and quality of life.

If you have a lot of weight to lose, don't let the amount frighten you or make you procrastinate. It took you some time to get to this stage in your life, and it's logical that it should take some time to get you back to normal.

HOW QUICKLY CAN YOU EXPECT TO LOSE WEIGHT?

Let's say you weigh 245 pounds. At an earlier time in your life you were comfortable at 185, and so a 60-pound weight loss would not seem out of the question. Here's a typical example of the progress that you should make, providing you adhere to the program. The first 30 pounds will come off in three to four months, giving you relief, more energy, and confidence that you can, in fact, do this. That would be reasonable. The last 30 pounds normally takes twice as long. Here's why. Before you begin the ONE**80** Plan, you weigh a lot and your body needs to burn a lot of calories just to keep going. You provide those calories with the foods you eat, so your weight stays the same. When you start the ONE**80** Plan, you begin taking in far fewer calories than your body needs to stay at that high weight, and so you lose weight, and pretty quickly too.

But after the first 30 pounds come off, your new body weighs much less than it did, and needs even fewer calories to maintain itself. You continue eating the same number of calories as in the first half of the Plan, however, the difference between what your body needs and what it is receiving is not as great as it was before, so you lose more slowly. So losing one pound or so per week (to get you back down to 185) will come in the second part of your weight loss.

Now, the overall weight loss may average out to a pound and a half per week. But when you arrive there, it will be easy for you to maintain, because you will have lost your weight eating in this healthy way. There is an added plus: the longer it takes you to lose, the more comfortable you will be with this new, healthy eating style that you have chosen for yourself. Always remember, you're not in a race. This time next year, you'll be one year older—and a lot thinner.

Everyone is different, and your rate of weight loss will vary depending on factors such as how closely you follow the food plan and whether or not you exercise. If you have any questions regarding whether you are losing weight at a safe rate, I strongly advise you to seek medical advice from your physician or health practitioner.

Let's move on to the plan itself—what you're going to eat, when, and how much.

WHAT ARE THE FIVE FOOD GROUPS?

If you're like most men, you know more about how your car works than you do about how your body works and how different foods affect your health. That's why your first step in the ONE**80** Plan is to learn what nutrients you need to be healthy, and what types of food to avoid. There are five food groups that, if eaten in the right proportions at the right time of day, will provide a healthy, balanced diet and never leave you hungry.

- The first group is vegetables and fruit.
- The second group is proteins, which includes meat, fish, cheese, legumes and eggs.
- The third group is grains and starches, which includes bread, cereal, pasta, rice, and potatoes.
- The fourth group is fats and oils.
- The fifth group is milk products, which includes milk and yoghurt.

Vegetables and Fruit

The first food group is vegetables and fruit. These foods contain vitamins, fiber, and minerals. They also contain antioxidants, which experts believe help protect us from heart disease and cancer, and protect our immune system. You probably have not been a big fruit and vegetable eater (which could be one reason for being overweight) and may not be aware of the wide choice of fresh varieties that are now available in your local supermarket.

Vegetables

Most vegetables can be eaten in unlimited quantities, anytime throughout the day. The more, the better! Vegetables are filled with nutrients that your body needs, and will allow you to fill up without taking in unnecessary calories. That's why I call them "anytime vegetables," and they're at the core of my ONE**80** Plan. There are many fresh and inter-esting varieties available, so you don't have to stick to lettuce and celery sticks. Carry a bag of peeled baby carrots with you in your car or keep some on hand in your desk or briefcase. Raw peppers or broccoli florets are delicious, and available in ready-to-eat packages at grocery stores.

Note that, in nutritional terms, potatoes are not considered a veg-etable. They are a starch, so make sure you include potatoes in your allocation for starches. The other exception is the avocado, which is a high-fat vegetable and should be considered a fat. You will see in my plan that I split vegetables into two categories—"anytime" because they contain virtually no calories and you can therefore fill up on them whenever you like, and "dinner" vegetables, which are higher in calo-ries and will make you more satisfied.

Fruit

Fruit should be your new snack because it can be eaten anywhere, anytime. You should have at least three helpings daily, beginning at breakfast. The fiber from fruit fills you up and keeps your hunger at bay for much longer than the donut, muffin, or bag of chips you used to grab on the way to work or at the vending machine. Having an apple mid-afternoon will satisfy your hunger in 10 minutes and stave off hunger for up to an hour.

Keep in mind that juice and dried fruits, such as raisins and dried cranberries, are higher in sugar than fresh fruit, so you should have smaller quantities of these foods. They're good for occasional treats. When you consider that one small box of raisins is equal, calorie-wise, to one apple, wouldn't you much rather eat a crisp, juicy apple? And a four-ounce glass of orange juice is equal to one orange or half a grape-fruit, and it doesn't provide you with the same fiber.

Proteins

Protein is essential to many bodily functions, and in my program it is included in every meal. Protein breaks down slowly and is digested over a long period of time, which makes you feel full for longer. For men, this is particularly important.

Proteins consist of up to 20 different amino acids; these help to build and repair tissue, including bones and muscles. They are also essential to cognitive function and memory. For this reason it is especially important to include protein in your breakfast—it will make you alert and active, and keep you feeling full right through until lunch.

You can get protein from different sources, and the type of protein that you eat is important.

Animal Protein

Animal protein is found in red meat, poultry, seafood, cheese, and eggs. Choose lean, trimmed cuts of red meat and low-fat, skinless poultry whenever possible. As with the section on vegetables, I choose to split proteins into two categories, high and low, because of the different calorie content. All types of fish are healthy and good choices. Another good source of protein is Omega eggs, which are healthier than regular eggs. Egg whites—whether you buy them as "egg beaters" at the grocery store or separate the eggs yourself—are a good and low-calorie substitute for whole eggs, since most of the fat in an egg is found in the yolk. High-fat cheese, which most cheese is, should be avoided or restricted. Hard cheeses contain a high amount of fat, and men tend to eat their cheese by the fistful, not as a nibble. So this will be an important change in your eating habits. There are now a number of cheeses that contain only five percent fat. Aim to switch to these low-fat alternatives. You will not find low-fat cheese in restaurants, so avoid ordering foods that contain cheese while you're out, and count on eating cheese only when you can get the low-fat variety from the supermarket.

Vegetable Protein

Vegetable protein is found in legumes, such as lentils, kidney beans, and chick peas, as well as in soya (found in tofu and other soya-based meat substitutes), and in grains like quinoa. Legumes are the ultimate protein because they are low in fat and high in fiber.

Grains and Starches

Grains and starches are an excellent source of energy, fiber, vitamins, and minerals. They also contain antioxidants. This food group will also be included in every meal.

You should pay close attention to the type of starches that you eat. Avoid white flour breads and choose whole wheat breads instead. Avoid white rice and choose brown or wild rice instead. For pastas, if a whole wheat variety is available, this is preferable. White flour and white grains have been highly processed to give them a longer shelf life, but the processing also removes some fiber and nutrients, such as iron and many B vitamins. The processing also makes these foods easier to digest, but the more quickly you digest your food, the more quickly your hunger returns. That leads you to eat more, because you are not satisfied. That's why the bread basket at dinner time is problematic. It fills you up quickly but sets you up for cravings for the rest of the meal.

There are lots of nutritious grains at your grocery store that are as easy to make as rice. Quinoa and amaranth are good examples. In the ONE**80** Plan, you'll be trying one new food each week, so it might be worth an extra five minutes in the grains aisle to experiment with new and delicious foods that you'd never thought of trying before.

Fats and Oils

The fourth group is fats and oils. We need some fat in our diet to carry out important bodily functions, and fat also provides energy. Your brain needs fats to function properly. And certain fats may improve your mood and your memory.

But because fats are "hidden" in so many prepared foods, it's easy to get too much of them. Fats are also dense calories: one gram of fat equals nine calories, but one gram of a protein or starch equals only four calories. Think about a Caesar salad: it starts with a plate of romaine lettuce (about 50 calories), but once the dressing (almost all fat) is added, your salad now contains about 1,500 calories. That dressing might not look like much, but it packs a calorie punch. (I call Caesar salad "lettuce leaves covered in fat.")

"Bad" Fats

These are the ones that increase our risk of coronary heart disease and provide no health benefit. These fats clog up our arteries because they increase LDL cholesterol levels, which is the "bad" cholesterol.

Bad fats are saturated fats that come from animal fat, such as butter and lard (and even hard cheeses). In general, if a fat is solid at room temperature, you know it's a bad fat.

Trans fats are also bad fats. A trans fat is a hydrogenated plant oil. Hydrogenation is a process developed in the early 1900s to prevent fats from becoming rancid. It extends the shelf life of oils and many other foods, but it also changes the molecular properties of the fat—to the detriment of our health. Trans fats are found in commercially prepared fried foods, processed foods and snack foods, prepared baked goods, peanut butter, and margarine.

There have been many articles written about trans fats in recent years because of their proven risk for heart disease. The city of New York recently went so far as to ban the use of trans fats in all its restaurants! Reading labels on food is so important: you have to know what you're putting into your body. The best medical advice is to eliminate trans fats from your diet, and that's what we advise with the ONE**80** Plan.

"Good" Fats

"Good" fats have a beneficial impact on cholesterol. These fats come in two categories: monounsaturated or polyunsaturated. Both are good for your heart because they boost HDL cholesterol, the "good" type. Unlike trans fats, good fats have not been modified from their natural state.

Monounsaturated fats are found in olive oil, canola oil, and peanut oil. (People in Mediterranean areas have a lower incidence of heart disease, possibly because they cook with olive oil instead of the hydrogenated cooking oil so popular in North America.) Polyunsaturated fats are found in vegetable oils like sunflower, corn, safflower, and soybean. Omega-6 and omega-3 polyunsaturated fats are also found in seafood, especially salmon, halibut, tuna, sardines, and mackerel, which are fatty cold-water fish.

The important thing to remember about fat intake is that you want to reduce it, not eliminate it. Instead of fearing all fats, eat only the amount that is recommended on the ONE**80** Plan.

Milk

Milk and dairy products are the fifth group. They are high in calcium, which is important for bone strength and preventing osteoporosis. Osteoporosis is softening of the bones. While it is more prevalent in older women than men, one in 10 men suffer from it. When you choose your dairy food, you should look for lower-fat alternatives, such as skim milk, low-fat or no-fat yoghurt, and low-fat cheese.

OTHER IMPORTANT COMPONENTS OF NUTRITION

Fiber

Fiber is a major factor in my ONE**80** Plan. It fills you up (remember satiety?), which will keep you from feeling hungry again soon after eating. Fiber cleans out your digestive tract, and it helps to control cholesterol levels by cleaning out the arterial areas. A high-fiber diet will help to lower your risk for colon cancer and heart disease.

Fiber is found in legumes, in grain foods such as whole wheat, wheat bran, and oat bran, and in many fruits and vegetables. When you increase the fiber in your diet, you will quickly notice that you are feeling "cleaner inside"; your bowel movements will become easier. Fiber is not a new thing. (Our grandparents referred to it as "bulk.")

Our digestive system needs a constant flow of fiber; it's both natural and necessary.

Reduced Salt

Much like fat, salt is essential for health but it's easy to get too much. Salt is especially harmful to people with high blood pressure or heart, liver, or kidney diseases. The U.S. Food and Drug Administration guideline is 2,400 mg of sodium per day—which is only one teaspoon.

The key to watching your salt levels is to be aware of foods that have a high sodium content. Check the nutrition labels of packaged foods, and be aware that frozen foods and processed foods, such as canned soup and canned vegetables, tend to have a high level of sodium (salt is used as a preservative). And you don't need a doctorate in food science to know that products like pretzels and potato chips are very high in salt content.

Keep your sodium intake within a healthy range by:

· Limiting your use of the salt shaker.
· Substituting salt seasoning with other flavorings, such as onion, garlic, lemon, vinegar, black pepper, or parsley. Or choose salt substitutes, which are available in your local grocery store.
· Watch the sodium content in your favorite condiments, especially soya sauce, steak sauce, ketchup, and salsa. Limit your intake accordingly.
· Beware of snack foods. One 10-ounce bag of Doritos contains over 1,500 milligrams of salt.
· Avoid foods with MSG (monosodium glutamate), particularly when dining out. You can ask to have your meal prepared without MSG.

GETTING STARTED ON THE ONE80 PLAN

The ONE80 Plan is simple to follow. Every food has a "unit value." The unit value depends on the food's calories, fiber, and fat. Unit values help you measure your food intake in the easiest possible fashion. The program outlines exactly how many units you can eat throughout the day, and also specifies the food type for each unit so that you are sure to meet all your nutritional needs.

The ONE**80** Plan is designed to allow you to choose from a broad range of foods, while encouraging a well-balanced, nutritionally sound program that meets both the Canada Food Guide and USDA Food Guide Pyramid. The program is based on eating highly nutritious foods that are low in calories, which is essential for you to lose weight. By sticking to a set number of units per day, you'll be able to achieve your goals.

There are three key rules to always keep in mind:

1. Stay with your **daily unit target**. You can't "bank" units or carry them forward to the next meal or the next day.
2. Follow the guidelines for **every type of unit** needed for each meal of the day. Do not skip any meals or shortchange the portion amounts for the food groups.
3. Every day, **use your daily eating awareness record** to plan what you will eat for each meal, including unit values. At the end of the day, track and record what you actually ate.

How Many Units Can I Eat?

The basic program is the same for everyone:

	Number and type of units per day
BREAKFAST (4 units)	2 protein 2 grain
LUNCH (4 units)	2 protein 2 grain
DINNER (7 units)	5 protein 1 starch 1 dinner vegetable
ANYTIME (5 units)	3 fruit 1 milk 1 fat
PLUS (0 units)	Anytime vegetables as desired Free selections as desired 8–12 glasses of water
Subtotal	**20 units per day**

This makes the ONE**80** Plan so easy to use. You'll find a list of foods and their unit values below, and you simply mix and match. For example, at breakfast, you need to have two units of protein and two units of grain. Perhaps you will choose to have two scrambled eggs with two ounces of whole wheat toast. You can add lettuce and tomato (Anytime Vegetables), as well as herbs and spices for flavor (Free Units). Of course, you'll want to have a glass of water, and if you are a coffee drinker, that is considered a free unit as well. You can also take from your Anytime Units and help yourself to an apple.

Later on you will see that I have provided you with an extensive list of foods and their unit values by category. To create your meals, all you need to do is look under each category and choose the food that you want to eat, determining the amount by the number of units that you're allowed in the chart. You'll find it easy to combine your new meals, and they will help you to stay full while losing extra pounds. Also at the end of the book I have provided you with an entire week's worth of recipes, all perfectly balanced for the ONE**80** Plan.

Additional Units

Because each man is unique, the ONE**80** Plan allows for additional units that tailor your program to suit your starting point. You don't have to use these extra units, but they are available to you if you find you are hungry or wanting something extra at one of your meals.

Sanity Savers

These foods and drinks are exactly what they are called. They are in the plan to give you relief when you are feeling hungry or are enjoying a social event. One of the best choices is air-popped popcorn. You can also have nachos with salsa, low-fat pretzels, or low-fat crackers; there are numerous kinds in your grocery store.

The number of additional units, replacement units, and sanity savers in your own program will depend on which of three entry levels you fall into. Answer these questions to determine your entry level.

Discover Which Program Is Right for You

Please answer each of the following questions yes or no.

Then add up the number of times you answered yes.

This will direct your selection of your entry level to start your ONE**80** Plan.

	YES	NO
1. Have you been overweight since age 10?	☐	☐
2. Have you been overweight since age 15?	☐	☐
3. Have you been overweight since age 20?	☐	☐
4. Have you been overweight since age 25?	☐	☐
5. Have you been overweight since age 30?	☐	☐
6. Have you been overweight since age 35?	☐	☐
7. Have you been overweight since age 40?	☐	☐
8. Do you have 25 lbs. or more to lose?	☐	☐
9. Do you have 40 lbs. or more to lose?	☐	☐
10. Do you have 60 lbs. or more to lose?	☐	☐
11. Do you have 80 lbs. or more to lose?	☐	☐
12. Do you have 100 lbs. or more to lose?	☐	☐
13. Do you have 125 lbs. or more to lose?	☐	☐
14. Is (or was) your father overweight?	☐	☐
15. Is (or was) your mother overweight?	☐	☐
16. Have you been continuously attempting various weight loss programs?	☐	☐
17. Do you find yourself eating after supper?	☐	☐
18. Do you find yourself eating late into the night?	☐	☐
19. Do you find yourself eating until you are stuffed?	☐	☐
20. Do you consider yourself a large protein eater? (Meats, poultry, hard cheese, fish, etc.)	☐	☐
21. Do you consider yourself a large fat eater? (Oils, butter, margarine, sauces, mayonnaise, etc.)	☐	☐
22. Do you dislike most types of fruits and vegetables?	☐	☐
23. Would you consider yourself a non-exercise person?	☐	☐
24. Is your workday primarily spent sitting?	☐	☐
25. Are there certain times in the day when you are overwhelmed by the desire for sweets?	☐	☐
TOTAL		

SELECT YOUR ENTRY LEVEL

1–7	"yes" answers	Level 1 ☐
8–16	"yes" answers	Level 2 ☐
17–25	"yes" answers	Level 3 ☐

Based on your entry level, you may now review the chart below to determine how many extra units per day you may eat.

	Level 1	Level 2	Level 3
ADDITIONAL UNITS	**2 additional units per day (if needed)** from any of these categories: · Protein · Fruit · Milk · Dinner vegetable · Sanity Saver (maximum 1) · Grain or starch (maximum 1) · Fat (maximum 1)	**4 additional units per day (if needed)** from any of these categories: · Protein · Fruit · Milk · Dinner vegetable · Sanity Savers (maximum 2) · Grains or starches (maximum 2)	**6 additional units per day (if needed)** from any of these categories: · Protein · Fruit · Milk · Dinner vegetable · Sanity Savers (maximum 2) · Grains or starches (maximum 2) · Fat (maximum 1)
Grand Total	**22 units per day**	**24 units per day**	**26 units per day**

Please Note: Throughout your weight loss:
If you are in level 1, you may stay at that level, or alternate between level 1 and level 2 after 45 days.
If you are in level 2, you may stay at that level or alternate with level 1.
If you are in level 3, you may alternate with level 1 or level 2 as desired.

How Much Is One Unit?

The following tables show how much of each food type equals one unit. Just choose what you like and create your own daily food plan. By following your daily unit targets, you'll find that you easily and automatically make great food choices that will help you to lose weight. The aim of the program is to choose foods that will make you feel full and satisfied, instead of consuming empty calories that give you no energy.

You will notice that there are two protein categories. I call one low category protein, and the other high category protein. I've put some restrictions on the number of times per week that you can eat from the high category protein list. You will also notice that I have identified two types of vegetables, "anytime vegetables" and "dinner vegetables." Anytime vegetables, of course, can be had whenever you like and as much as you like. However, dinner vegetables should only be eaten with dinner.

All weights are to be measured after cooking and, in the case of protein, with bones removed.

PROTEIN

Low Category Protein

Dairy (Each of the amounts below = 1 unit)

Cottage Cheese 2 oz.	1 medium egg or 2 tbsp. of egg whites
Hard Cheese (low fat – 1% – 2%) 1 oz.	(6 eggs per week)
Ricotta Cheese (low fat – 5%) 1 oz.	

Fish (with less than 20% fat; 1 oz. cooked = 1 unit)

Arctic Char	Monk Fish
Brook Trout	Perch
Cod	Pike
Flounder	Red Snapper
Grouper	Scrod
Haddock	Sea Bass
Halibut	Sole
Mahi Mahi	Tuna (water packed)

Shellfish (1 oz. cooked = 1 unit)

Clams	Scallops
Crab	Shrimp
Lobster	Squid
Mussels	

Meat (1 oz. cooked = 1 unit)

Chicken	Turkey Breast
Game – Venison, Rabbit	

All Legumes (½ cup = 1 unit)

Chick Peas	Lentils
Kidney Beans	Lima Beans

High Category Protein: *Restrict to twice per week, preferably at breakfast or lunch, and once per week for dinner*

Dairy

Higher fat cheese (15% fat content) (1 oz. = 1 unit)
Hard cheese
Feta cheese

Fish with more than 20% fat (1 oz. cooked = 1 unit)

Black Sea Bass	Shark
Lox	Smoked Salmon
Mackerel	Swordfish
Orange Ruffi	Trout (lake, ocean, rainbow)
Polok Fish	Tuna (oil packed)
Salmon	Turbot
Sardines (water packed)	White Fish

Meats (1 oz. cooked = 1 unit)

Beef (Lean)	Pork
Lamb	Tongue
Liver	Veal
Hot Dogs (All Beef, Veal, Turkey or Chicken)	

Miscellaneous (Each of the amounts below = 1 unit)
Tofu – 1oz.
Peanut Butter – 1 tbsp.
Whey Protein – 1oz.

GRAIN AND STARCH (1 oz. = 1 unit)

Whole Grain Bread
4 Melba Toast Rectangles
6 Melba Toast Rounds
Whole Grain English Muffin
Whole Wheat Pita
Rolls
Raisin Bread
Bagels
Rolls
1 80-calorie portion specialty cracker (e.g., Ryvita, Wasa, Kavli)
1 Board Matzo
2 Rice Cakes
Cooked hot cereal – ½ cup
Cold unsugared cereal – 1 oz.
Unprocessed bran – ¼ cup
Whole Wheat Pasta – ½ cup cooked
Brown or Wild Rice – ½ cup cooked
Baked Potato – 1 small
Couscous – ½ cup cooked

FRUIT (Average size = 1 unit)

1 Apple, medium
3 Apricots
Banana (small – 4 oz.)
½ cup Blackberries
½ cup Blueberries
½ Cantaloupe, small
10 Cherries
3 Dates
2 Figs
½ cup unsweetened Fruit Juice
½ cup Fruit packed in unsweetened juice
½ medium Grapefruit
½ cup Grapes
2-inch wedge (1 cup) Honeydew Melon
2 Kiwi
3 small Mandarins

½ Mango
1 medium Nectarine
1 medium Orange
½ medium Papaya
1 medium Peach
1 small Pear
1 medium Persimmon
¼ fresh Pineapple
½ cup Pineapple (packed in its own juice)
2 small Plums
3 Prunes
⅓ cup Prune Juice
½ cup Raspberries
1 cup Strawberries
1 medium Tangerine
1 cup Watermelon

ANYTIME VEGETABLES (unlimited quantities)

Asparagus
Bamboo Shoots
Bok Choy
Broccoli
Brussels Sprouts
Cabbage
Carrots
Cauliflower
Celery
Cucumber
Dill Pickle
Dill Tomatoes
Eggplant
Endive
Lettuce
Mushrooms
Onions, raw
Parsley

Peppers
Pimento
Radicchio
Radishes
Rappini
Rhubarb
Sauerkraut
Scallions
Spinach
Sprouts
String Beans
Summer Squash
(Vegetable Marrow,
Spaghetti squash)
Tomato
Turnip
Zucchini

DINNER VEGETABLES (½ cup cooked = 1 unit)

Artichokes
Beets
Corn, canned
Corn, fresh, ½ ear
Leeks
Mixed Vegetables
Okra
Onions, cooked
Parsnip
Peas

Pumpkin
Rutabaga
Snow Peas
Squash
(Acorn, Butternut
Hubbard, Pepper)
Tomato Sauce or Spaghetti Sauce
Water Chestnut
½ medium Yam

FAT (each of the quantities below = 1 unit)

1 tsp. Margarine
1 tsp. Diet Margarine
1 tsp. Butter
1 tsp. Oil (monounsaturated preferred)
1 tsp. Mayonnaise
2 tsp. Lite Mayonnaise
2 tsp. Salad Dressing
2 tbsp. Cream, 10%
1 tbsp. Cream Cheese
2 tbsp. Lite Cream Cheese

MILK (1 unit per day) each of the quantities below = 1 unit
Low-fat or Zero-fat selections always preferred.
1 cup Skim Milk
¾ cup low fat plain Yoghurt
1 cup Buttermilk
½ cup evaporated Skim Milk
1 serving calorie reduced Cocoa mix
½ cup 2% Milk
¾ cup 1% Milk

FREE UNITS (as desired)
Water (min. 8–12 glasses daily)

Herbs & Spices	Pepper
Paprika	Salt
Coffee (decaf. preferred)	Tea (herbal)
Pan Spray	Vinegar
Artificial Sweetener	Soy Sauce
Diet Beverages	Lime
Bouillon	Horseradish
Tamari Sauce	Diet Jell-O

Worcestershire Sauce
Lemon
Mustard
Clear Soup (fat-free)
1 tbsp. Diet Salad Dressing (per day)
2 tsp. Ketchup (per day)
2 tsp. Diet Jam (per day)
2 tsp. Diet Maple Syrup (per day)
1 tsp. Cocoa (per day)
1 tbsp. Grated Cheese (per day)

SANITY SAVERS

1 tbsp. Tartar Sauce	2 tbsp. Barbecue Sauce
2 tbsp. Teriyaki Sauce	2 tbsp. Relish
2 tbsp. Cranberry Sauce	½ cup Seafood Cocktail Sauce
2 cups plain Popcorn	3 cups air-popped Popcorn
1 oz. Nachos	1 oz. low-fat Pretzels
2 tbsp. Corn Starch	2 tbsp. Flour
1 oz. Raisins	¼ medium Avocado
¼ cup Baked Beans	½ cup Frozen Yoghurt
½ cup Ice Milk	1 oz. Liquor
8 oz. Beer	12 oz. Lite Beer
4 oz. Wine (red or white, dry)	4 oz. Champagne

Note: If a food is not on the list (for example, chocolate cake), it's because I believe that you cannot allow yourself to eat this and expect to lose weight. This is also true for mixed dishes like lasagna which can vary dramatically in the number of units, depending on the recipe.

Food-preparation Guidelines

· Weigh all foods. Weigh proteins and grains after cooking.

· Broil, boil, bake, steam, or roast. You may use cooking spray for frying, but never use other fats for frying. Do not deep fry.

· Remove all visible fat from meat before cooking, and remove poultry and fish skin before eating.

· Count any milk used in coffee, tea, or cereal as part of your daily allowance.

How to Plan Your Meals

I encourage you to plan your own meals and to create as much variety within the program as you like. Most of my clients get into a routine of what they enjoy and stick with it from week to week.

However, some people like to start with a suggested menu, and so later in the chapter I have provided one as an example.

Plan your snacks. This is important if you are to keep to the program. Try low-fat crackers, air-popped popcorn, low-fat pretzels, or frozen yoghurt in addition to fruit and vegetables.

DAILY EATING AWARENESS RECORD

As you now know, research shows that keeping track of what you eat gives you better weight loss success. Even if you think you have a great memory, you'd be surprised at how easy it is to forget those little additions throughout the day — milk in your coffee, or a piece of cheese on your sandwich. Studies suggest that when people report their own caloric intake, without having a written record, they significantly underestimate their consumption of high-calorie foods and overestimate the low-calorie foods. The *only* way to assess how many units you eat each day is by making a record. It will do wonders to help you become aware of the foods you're eating and how often, and will give you insight as to why you may be eating them.

Below, you will find a sample of a daily eating awareness record that comes directly from one of my clients. It is simple to use and will help you to organize all your information so you can compare days quickly and easily. You will see that it also has a place for you to indicate what exercise you have done on that day, and how you are feeling. You may download samples of the form by going to itsdifferentformen. com, or by turning to page 132 and photocopying the Daily Eating Awareness Record.

Daily Eating Awareness Record

Name: _John Doe_

Week of: _January 15, 2008_

Action Steps This Week

1. _Buy new running shoes_

2. _Try Tilapia fish_

3. _Plan business lunch with Mark_

Lost this week: _2.5_ lbs

Lost to date: _30_ lbs

Week #: _11_

Please remember to log your daily feelings along with what you eat.

Codes
GR – great   VS – very strong
G – good   OK – okay

Maximum: Eggs – 6/wk
Hard cheese –4 ox/wk

Breakfast	2 Slices, 9 Grain Toast, 1
6:30 am	poached Omega Egg, 2 oz FF Cot Cheese, 1/2 C Skim Milk
Snack	
10:00 am	Peach
Lunch	
12:00 pm	2 slices Whole grain Bread, 2 oz Tuna, Lettuce Salad/Dr
Snack	
3:00 pm	Apple
Dinner	5 oz Barbequed Strip Loin Steak,
5:45 pm	Baked Potato, Lettuce Salad/Dr, 1/2 C Corn, 1/2 C Skim Milk
Snack	
10:30 pm	1/2 C Fat Free Yogurt, 1/2 C Grapes
Drinks	

Daily Checklist

Water	⊙⊙⊙⊙⊙⊙⊙⊙⊙○○
Protein	⊙⊙⊙⊙⊙⊙⊙⊙
Grain/Starch	⊙⊙⊙⊙⊙
Fruit ⊙⊙⊙	Fat ⊙○○ Milk ⊙○○
Dinner Veg ⊙	Anytime Veg ⊙⊙
Additional Units ○○○○○○	

Exercise	Time: _9:00_ (am/pm)
YES/No?	Duration _30_ (min)
Activity:	_Speed Walking_

Daily Feelings (circle one)

GR   VS   G   OK

Progress Notes:
Feel like I'm on track

Success Guidelines

- Read the program over again several times to make sure that you thoroughly understand how it works.
- Follow the program exactly as written for best results.
- Discuss your new plan with those around you who may be of assistance in your project.

- Food planning should be an active practice rather than a passive one. It is most important that you learn to anticipate all outside-the-home eating situations.
- Always shop by list and leave nothing to chance.
- Read all labels.

A Typical Day

Breakfast: Two ounces of whole wheat bread with two poached eggs plus a half a grapefruit and a cup of coffee or tea. Or, 1 ounce of cold cereal with a small sliced banana, 8 ounces of skim milk, plus a half a cup of cottage cheese and one slice of whole wheat bread. Or, on the run, a pack of melba toast and two hard-boiled eggs in the car.

Always consider including a unit of fruit. By adding a banana or berries to your cereal, you are adding fiber to your diet; we've already discussed the importance of fiber for the smooth functioning of your digestive system.

The mid-morning snack: At about 10:30 a.m. try some water and an apple.

Lunch: Lunch should not be so filling that you find yourself fatigued due to the heavy calories, but it must be filling enough to pacify your hunger.

Take two slices of bread, wrapped separately, with the filler (perhaps tuna or two hard boiled eggs or sliced cooked turkey or chicken) and place them in a large plastic airtight container mixed with a generous portion of your favorite "anytime vegetables." Always feel free to pile veggies like cucumber slices, sprouts, or tomatoes on your open-faced sandwich. But do not have mayonnaise on your sandwich. Replace it with mustard and cut out one unit of fat!

In restaurants, when on business or alone, it is best to concentrate on salads. If you choose a salad, eat one that has crunchy vegetables, not just lettuce, which is mostly water. You need food that has fiber, which will fill you up.

Many restaurants feature grilled chicken or grilled shrimp or tuna or even poached salmon. If you are able to get your protein on top of your favorite salad, go for it. You will even have room to add a two-ounce bagel or a whole wheat bun on the side. Remember to use a knife and fork: you will find yourself eating slower and more conscientiously. You may include half a cantaloupe or a sugar-free fruit cup at lunch as well.

The mid-afternoon snack: About 3:30 or 4:00 most men experience an energy dip because they are hungry. Have a fruit or raw vegetables, like peeled carrots that come pre-packaged.

Dinner: Dinner calls for five protein units, vegetables, and starch. The starch, which is potatoes, pasta, or rice, is included at dinner because it is the food that you need to carry you forward for the longest time . . . until breakfast. It will ensure that you do not go to bed feeling ravenous. There is no bread at dinner. It's best to get used to not eating bread in the evening. The temptation when dining out is to reach for the bread basket. This is a habit that you must break.

The evening meal for most men should be a good size, filled with low-fat vegetables as well as a starch and a portion of protein. A five-ounce portion of chicken breast is a low-fat staple for many of my clients. Seasoned to your own taste, it is easy to get in any restaurant and quick to make at home on your barbecue or grill. Have a baked potato as your starch and sprinkle some lemon juice on it. Steamed vegetables may be had in large quantities except for the dinner vegetable (higher-sugar vegetables). Mix corn kernels ("dinner vegetable") with string beans, or any other "anytime vegetable."

Also at dinner you can stir-steam your veggies with soy and water together with a five-ounce portion of shrimp. Place it on a bed of brown rice. Be sure to leave the table satisfied and in the evening have some popcorn from the "Sanity Savers List" or some fruit with yoghurt.

SAMPLE MENU PLAN

Breakfast

Stick-to-your-ribs breakfast

- 2 Grain –1 cup hot oatmeal
- 2 Protein – ½ cup low-fat cottage cheese
- 1 Fruit – 1 medium peach (or ½ cup tinned, packed in its own juice)
  Peel and slice the peach to mix with the cottage cheese.

Lunch

Turkey sandwich

- 2 Protein – 2 oz. lean, sliced deli turkey
- 2 Grain – 1 small whole wheat bagel
- Anytime Vegetable – sliced tomato and cucumber, shredded lettuce, dill pickle (optional)
- Anytime Vegetable – bagged coleslaw mix drizzled with apple cider vinegar
- Sanity Saver – ¼ medium avocado
- 1 Fruit – 1 medium peach

Dinner

Salmon with herbs

- 5 Protein – 5 oz. salmon filet
- 1 clove garlic, minced
- ¼ cup chopped fresh dill or ½ tsp. dried dill
- 1 Starch – 1 small baked potato with salsa
- 1 Dinner Vegetable – ½ cup corn niblets, cooked
- 1 Fat – 1 tsp. of margarine
- Free – 1 cup chicken broth
- Anytime Vegetable – chopped carrots, celery, zucchini, and tomatoes added to the chicken broth
- 1 Fruit – 2 wedges (1 cup) honeydew melon

Preparation

Preheat oven to 450 degrees. Sprinkle salmon with garlic and dill. Bake 7 to 10 minutes depending on thickness of filet. Fish is done when it flakes easily with fork. Do not overcook!

TIPS FOR PLANNING A WEEKLY MENU

Here are some guidelines on how to plan your own menus. One of the best ways to ensure that you stick to my ONE**80** Plan is to be prepared: set aside time each week—before going to the grocery store—to plan a menu for the next seven days. You can choose from the menu plan and from the recipes at the end of the book or make up your own. From this plan, you can create a shopping list. The more times you do this, the more it will become routine. With experience, menu planning takes less than half an hour of your time.

· Keep the menus practical and simple. But, at the same time, don't exclude good flavor and fun. Remember that you need to enjoy your meals if you're expecting to stick with your plan.

· For breakfast and lunch, you must eat proteins and grains. This combination helps suppress your hunger and stimulates your brain. This is very important because most men like to skip breakfast, or buy a muffin on the way to the office, and often skimp on lunch, or miss it altogether. Lunch should be fulfilling and satisfying but not to the point of the mid-afternoon slump from overeating. No matter how pressed you are for time, don't skip lunch; you'll only be more tempted to eat later in the day when your energy level nosedives. The result is that you become so ravenous by the middle of the afternoon you grab whatever is handy, like a bag of chips or a chocolate bar, and then continue to remain hungry for the rest of the day. This brings on the night eating, after having a big dinner. Does this pattern sound familiar?

· Plan your snacks. This is important if you are to keep to the program. Try low-fat crackers, air-popped popcorn, low-fat pretzels, or frozen yoghurt in addition to fruit and vegetables.

- Aim for variety. Try new fruits and vegetables. Be sure to buy them for snacks as well as for your meals. Try legumes. Look up some fantastic and easy recipes at the end of the book or go to www. itsdifferentformen.com for a greater selection. These are filling and delicious. Buy spices to enhance the flavor of your food.
- Don't make meat the focus. Build the main part of your meal around vegetables and fruits, in addition to rice, noodles, or other grains.
- Have fun. Some of your planning efforts may at first seem like number-crunching in order to get to the exact number of units. But don't forget that good and healthy food is one of life's pleasures. Take advantage of flavors, colors, and textures to create enticing dishes. A varied selection of foods helps delight the senses. Include your favorites. It's okay to include your favorite foods in your weekly menus on occasion, though you may need to adapt recipes to make them healthier. Look for ways to reduce the fat and calories without significantly affecting the taste or texture (e.g., replacing cream with low-fat milk, using a lean cut of meat instead of a high-fat cut).
- A word about dairy. The plan allows one unit of dairy for milk in your coffee or with your cereal. You can also have low-fat yoghurt as a snack. After-dinner yoghurt is a favorite with many men.
- Remember the importance of water. Drinking eight to 12 glasses of water each day is an important step in helping to curb your hunger. Quite often, men mistake thirst for hunger. Water will quench your thirst and keep you from eating when you are not really hungry.
- The combination of sugar and chocolate—the candy bar—has done untold damage to North American waistlines. It is the pairing of fat, which is high in calories, and caffeine in the chocolate that wreaks havoc. The caffeine is very addictive and you always want more. You can't stop at a couple of bites. The same is true for soda drinks; cut them out immediately. Try to replace them with water, which you can flavor with lime or lemon. If this is too traumatic, switch to diet soda and try to gradually replace it with water.

Quick Reference: Your Weekly Menu

	Eat Regularly	Don't Eat
Cooking method	Steam, bake, or grill your meat & fish	Fried in hydrogenated, palm, or coconut oil, batter crust, deep fried (e.g., chicken wings)
Grains & starch – breads, pasta, & rice	Whole wheat bread & pasta, brown or wild rice, baked potato	French fries
Toppings & sauces	Mustard, low-fat margarine, tomato-based sauces, yoghurt dips, lemon juice & herbs, sodium-reduced soy sauce, vinegars	Mayonnaise, butter, cream-based sauces, gravy
Soups	Clear broth	Cream-based broth, chowders
Desserts	Fruit, low-fat yogurt, sugar-free applesauce, non-fat frozen yoghurt	Sweets with sugar, chocolate, cookies, doughnuts, pastries, muffins, cakes, cookies, pies, ice cream, candy bars
Snacks	Air-popped or plain popcorn, tortilla chips & salsa, nachos, low-fat pretzels, low-fat crackers, nuts—in controlled portions	Chips of any kind, pizza with cheese, chicken wings
Drinks	Lots of water, diet sodas, low-fat or skim milk, coffee (decaf preferred), tea (herbal preferred)	Regular soft drinks, flavored coffees, whole milk

HOW TO MAKE BETTER CHOICES

Paul's unit target is 22. For breakfast, Paul has been eating granola, OJ, and coffee, which equals a value of 11 units. With just a few simple changes, Paul can save 5 units.

Play with this yourself; it's easy to choose new, healthier replacements for your old habits. You now have a list of great foods to choose from, and you'll be surprised by how much more food you can eat when your choices are nutrient-dense and yet low in calories.

Paul's old choice	The better choice
8 grain units – 1 cup granola	1 grain unit – 1 oz. Shredded Wheat & Bran
2 fruit units – 8 oz orange juice	1 fruit unit – ½ cup blueberries
1 milk unit – ½ cup whole milk	1 milk unit – ¾ cup 1% milk
	1 grain unit – 1 oz. whole wheat bagel
	2 protein units – 2 oz. "La Vache Qui Rit" (68% less fat) cheese
free units – black coffee	free units – black coffee
11 units Total	**6 units Total**

WEIGH AND MEASURE YOURSELF ONCE EACH WEEK

In order to determine how you are doing, you have to keep track of your progress. This is an essential part of the program, and I'm very particular about how you do it. As I said before, don't jump on and off the scales every day.

You'll need to weigh yourself and measure your waist size once each week and record the results in your "Daily Eating Awareness Record" sheets; but remember, once you've picked the day of the week that you're going to do it, stick with that day and that day only. Don't do it more often, because your weight can easily fluctuate, and this can lead you to become discouraged or to relax your efforts—neither of which would be a good result.

For the most accurate results when weighing and measuring yourself:

· Use the same scale each week.
· Weigh and measure yourself at the same time of day each week.
· Wear similar clothes. If you wore shoes the first time, always wear shoes when you weigh yourself.
· To measure your waist circumference, take off your shirt and loosen your belt.
· Position the tape midway between the top of your hip bone and the bottom of your rib cage, usually at the level of your navel.

- Do not measure your waist where you wear your belt. Put the tape around your belly button.
- When taking your waist measurement, the abdomen should be relaxed and you should be breathing out.

On your weight-tracking day, enter your new weight and waist measurement into your daily eating awareness record. Check out your progress from the week before. Keep your weight information updated, so that you can track your improvement. If you've gained some weight, check back in your notes. What were you eating? See if your diet varied from other weeks when you were successful.

NOT QUITE "FOOD": ALCOHOL AND THE ONE80 PLAN

For many men, cutting alcohol consumption is one of the most effective ways to lose weight. If your drinking is not in moderation, you will not meet your weight loss goal. A moderate level is considered to be no more than two drinks per day. A drink is a 12-ounce bottle of beer, a 5-ounce glass of wine, or 1½ ounces of spirits.

While you don't have to stop drinking alcohol, if you want to lose weight, you have to keep your consumption in check. Alcohol is loaded with calories and has no nutritional value.

- Alcohol contains seven calories per gram.
- Protein provides four calories.
- Carbohydrate provides four calories.
- Fat provides nine calories.
  Even worse, many alcoholic cocktails also contain sugars.

The Other Disadvantages of Alcohol

There are a lot of other negatives involved in drinking too much:

- Too much alcohol will add fat to your waist size.
- Too much alcohol increases your risk of high blood pressure.

- It lessens your resolve to follow your new eating habits and lose the weight. If you drink before or during a meal, it lowers your inhibitions and willpower.
- Alcohol stimulates your appetite.
- It slows down the rate at which your body burns fat.
- It is a depressant and lowers your self-esteem.

Moreover, in socializing with your friends, many foods that accompany drinking (chips, peanuts, pretzels) are salty and make you thirsty, encouraging you to drink even more. To compensate, have some water between your drinks.

Skipping a meal to save your calories for drinks later—"banking" the calories—is tempting, but it's a bad move. If you come to the bar hungry, you are even more likely to munch on the snacks, and drinking on an empty stomach enhances the negative effects of alcohol.

Tips on How to Reduce Alcohol Consumption

Many men find reducing their alcohol level more difficult than changing their eating habits. If you are one of them, here are some tips on how to reduce your consumption.

1. Plan ahead for when someone offers you a drink and you will decline. Decide what you will say and write it down. Learn how to say NO. You do not have to drink when other people drink. You do not have to take a drink that is given to you. Practice ways to say no politely. For example, you can tell people you feel better when you drink less.
2. Increase the number of alcohol-free days you have each week. Many men find it helpful to avoid alcohol during the week and allow themselves a treat at weekends only. Pick a day or two each week when you will not drink at all. Then, try to stop drinking for one week. Think about how you feel physically and emotionally on these days. When you succeed and feel better, you may find it easier to cut down for good.
3. Reduce the amount of alcohol that you keep in your house. Don't keep temptations around.

4. Create a spritzer by mixing your wine with club soda or a mineral water.

5. Have a Virgin Mary or Caesar instead of the real thing.

6. Replace mixes with diet sodas. Make low-calorie choices. It's also important to choose your drinks sensibly (both from a calorie and alcohol-content point of view). For example, two single gin and slimline tonics provide just two units of alcohol and 100 calories, compared with two glasses of wine—four units of alcohol and 250 calories. Yet both take roughly the same amount of time to drink.

7. If you drink spirits at home, buy a measure and use it rather than pouring straight from the bottle.

8. When possible, plan to avoid situations where there will be pressure to drink a lot.

9. If you're planning on drinking later, eat a healthy meal first. You'll feel fuller, which will stop you from overdrinking.

10. Drink at least one glass of water before you start drinking. This will help quench your thirst and slow down the drinking.

11. Savor the taste of your drink. Put down your glass after each swallow. Extend the time between rounds of drinks.

12. Keep a diary of your drinking, just as you do for your food. You may be surprised. How different is your goal from the amount you drink now?

13. Try replacing drinking time with something fun with your family or friends. Use the time and money on something else. You'll feel much better.

14. Get support. Ask your family and friends for support to help you reach your goal. Drinking less will pay big dividends.

Units in Drinks

Beer: Raise Your Glass with Care

Beer is the next-best choice for dieters after a spritzer with about 140 calories per 12-ounce serving. Choosing light beers will drop your caloric intake without sacrificing much flavor, but keep in mind that it can be hard to estimate your intake when pouring from a pitcher or into an oversized beer mug.

Drink	Serving Size	Calories	Units
Red wine	5 oz.	100	1
White wine	5 oz.	100	1
Champagne	5 oz.	130	2
Light beer	12 oz.	105	1
Regular beer	12 oz.	140	2
Dark beer (lager)	12 oz.	170	2
Dark beer (ale)	1.5 oz.	82	1
Martini	1.5 oz.	100	1
Gin & Tonic	4 oz.	90	1
Rum & Soda	4 oz.	90	1
Margarita	4 oz.	100	1
Whiskey Sour	4 oz.	125	1
Liqueurs	1 oz.	100	1

MY ONE80 PLAN FOR LIFE SUCCESS

So there it is: my ONE80 Plan for men. I've used units instead of calories in order to create a program that is easy to follow yet still provides you with the tools to change your life. It is nutritious, and you can follow it anywhere you travel. It is also flexible enough that you can eat a wide variety of normal foods, and—of paramount importance—you will never be hungry.

I know taking away that hunger greatly reduces your temptation to fall off the wagon, which can be the pitfall for so many of us. It truly is a program designed for the rest of your life, and I know that you can and will use it to get control of your eating and move with confidence towards a future of health and success.

DAILY EATING AWARENESS RECORD

BREAKFAST
_____ a.m.

Snack
_____ a.m.

LUNCH
_____ a.m.

DINNER
_____ p.m.

Snack
_____ p.m.

Drinks

Daily Checklist
Water o o o o o o o o o o o o
Protein o o o o o o o o o
Grain/Starch o o o o o
Fruit o o o   Fat o o o   Milk o o o
Dinner Veg o Anytime Veg o o
Additional Units o o o o o o

Exercise   Time _____ (a.m./p.m.)
Yes/No?   Duration _____ (min.)
Activity: _____

Daily Feelings (circle one)
        GR   VS   G   OK
Progress Notes:
_____

SPORTS AND EXERCISE ARE NOT THE SAME THING

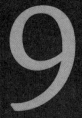

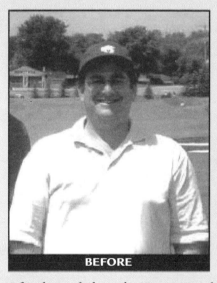

BEFORE

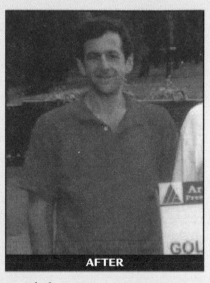

AFTER

I first learned about the Harvey Brooker weight loss program in 2003. I was a 44-year-old overweight man, facing a future of further weight gain. I decided it was time to take some action for my family and myself. Over the next eight months I lost 80 pounds and have maintained that weight loss for four years. I am healthy, active, and able to enjoy life and take part in activities with my children. My family and friends are still amazed at the change and I firmly believe this program has added years to my life.

Eric Cohen

We need to spend some time talking about exercise, because as you change your life you'll have to commit to it on a regular basis.

Exercise is absolutely vital to your health as you attempt to get to and maintain your ideal weight. It kick-starts the metabolism, increases muscle mass, gives more energy, and lays the groundwork for a more efficient and able body.

Regular physical activity is crucial to weight loss—and to maintaining that loss once you have taken the pounds off. Within weeks of becoming more active, you will notice that you have more energy, are in better spirits, sleep better, and simply find it easier to function. Physical activity decreases the stress that can lead to overeating. It also reduces appetite.

You may be concerned that you don't have the stamina to exercise, but it's just the opposite. Even a small amount of physical activity will give you more energy. Regular physical activity, especially if you include some strength training, not only burns calories but can build muscle. Muscle burns significantly more calories than body fat. A three-pound increase in the amount of muscle in your body can potentially burn enough extra calories to lose an additional 10 pounds over a year.

Start slowly, especially if you haven't exercised for a while. The good news: you don't have to be a jock to do it. Build up gradually so that you never risk any damage to your body (or your ego) in the process. Once you make exercise a part of your life, you'll discover it can be a pure delight and something you look forward to. The keys are to ease into it gradually, build up slowly, do it regularly, and vary what you do (so you won't get bored). It does get easier and the results will motivate you to make activity part of your everyday life.

Aim for 30 minutes of moderate physical activity most days of the week, preferably daily. Your program should also include aerobic exercises and stretching as well as exercises with weights to improve strength, two to three times per week.

GETTING STARTED

If you were a jock in your youth, I know what you're thinking. You'll just go back to playing pick up basketball or touch football with more regularity, right? If you're in the north, maybe you'll be saying that it's only a question of lacing up the skates for a few evenings a week.

But in fact, you must make a clear distinction between sport and exercise. As I said, exercise is vital to you. For the sake of my program, think of it as bodily exertion for the sake of improving your health. A sport, on the other hand, is a physical activity, perhaps competitive, played by a set of rules. When you engage in sport it may or may not involve the exertion that you ultimately need to improve your fitness.

Sport is fun, and depending on the sport it will get you moving to some degree; it will even burn some calories, depending on how vigorously you play and for how long. If you do strenuous sport frequently enough, it is a great way of getting your exercise, but it's also important to know that you can exercise without participating in sport at all, and that not all sports provide great exercise.

On the other hand, you may be thinking, "Oh my god, I'm not an athlete. What am I going to do?" Nobody wants to be the overweight guy surrounded by body builders at the gym.

Perhaps it's been some time since you took part in any activity. Maybe back in senior high? A report from the U.S. Centers for Disease Control indicated that 55 percent of American adults don't meet the minimum physical activity requirements (30 minutes of moderate activity on most days of the week). You're not alone!

There's no question that if you want to achieve a steady weight loss, then you need to get moving. But don't worry; a complicated, strenuous workout is not necessary when you start out. Instead, just head out for a 30 minute walk. The important thing to remember is the frequency of the activity.

In the long run, to get the maximum benefit, your exercise should consist of two elements. First and foremost, it should include aerobic and calorie-burning activities, such as walking, jogging, swimming, or bicycle riding. Second, you should introduce weight training, which offers many benefits, such as building muscle and strength, boosting immunity, and reducing the risk of low-back injury.

Choose an activity that you like and one you can keep on doing. And just keep going at a nice steady pace. Since your goal is frequency, you've got to choose an activity that is easy and enjoyable to do.

If you're out of shape, take it very easy while you build up your strength and endurance. And if you're really out of shape, you should consult your health care provider before embarking on an activity program.

Walking Off Calories

In order to lose weight and get yourself fitter and healthier, you need to build up to walking at least 10,000 steps a day—about five miles. With every five miles that you walk, you are actually burning off about 500 calories.

If you walk up an incline, the calories used will add up even faster. Just for fun, here is a list of how many steps it takes to burn off the calories in some classic "treats." Next time you want to avoid the temptation of that chocolate bar, remind yourself that you would need to add 2,393 steps to your daily routine just to stay in balance!

- A glass of red wine = 2,050 steps
- A rum and coke = 2,400 steps
- Just one ounce of potato chips = 3,300 steps
- A spring roll = 8,200 steps
- A bagel with cinnamon and raisins = 6,200 steps
- A portion of chocolate ice cream = 4,500 steps
- A large whole-milk latte = 5,450 steps
- A slice of pepperoni pizza = 5,000 steps
- A portion of Christmas pudding and brandy butter = 8,450 steps
- A pint of beer = 4,100 steps
- A large chocolate bar with nuts = 8,500 steps

- Two large chocolate chip cookies = 5,100 steps
- 2 ounces of cheddar cheese = 5,200 steps
- 3 ounces of white boiled rice = 2,200 steps
- A portion of roast chicken (no skin) = 4,150 steps
- A small carrot = 45 steps
- A cherry tomato = 14 steps

Get Walking

Getting started is easy. Simply increasing the amount of walking that you do is an easy and effective way for anyone to begin to get back into shape.

- Start out with 10 to 15 minutes per day for the first couple of weeks.
- Take the stairs instead of the elevator.
- Park the car at the far end of the parking lot so you have to walk to your destination, or get off the bus one stop earlier, so you have to walk.
- If you have an errand, walk to the corner store instead of driving.
- Take the dog out for an extra walk.

There is no need to complete your physical exercise all at one time. It can be spread over two or three times during the day. Set manageable goals for walking, and then gradually increase what I refer to as the three F's:

- Frequent: exercise more often.
- Further: slowly increase the distance you walk, run, or bike.
- Faster: slowly decrease the time that it takes you to walk, run, or bike the same distance.

Resistance Training

Along with your new routine of walking, you will be incorporating a short muscle-building workout with weights. A recent study published in the *American Journal of Cardiology* showed that a group of people who did a combination of resistance training and aerobic exercise had a tremendous increase in their overall endurance and strength as compared to a group that participated in only aerobic exercises.

Resistance training, or weight training, is probably the most neglected component of fitness programs, but it's one of the most beneficial. Muscle is metabolically active tissue. This means that it uses calories to work and to repair and refuel itself. Fat requires very few calories; it just kind of sits there. Every pound of muscle on your body takes up to 50 calories a day to maintain. A pound of fat only requires two calories a day to sustain it!

Weights are inexpensive and easy to use at home, and there are countless guidebooks and online resources with workouts for every level. If you'd rather get some one-on-one coaching, join your local gym. Most gyms will take you on a tour with a trainer and help you to create your own easy workout plan. Keep your routine quick and simple, and do it regularly.

Keep in mind that 30 minutes of moderate-intensity activity a day is an excellent starting point, not an upper limit. Exercising longer, or harder, or both, can bring even greater health benefits. There is now well-documented evidence of the benefits of hard exercise in terms of its ability to slow down or reverse aging.

Once you've built a routine and some stamina, you can start to add some variety into your activity in order to keep up your interest and build even more endurance. Cross-country ski, jog, or swim. It's your choice. Joining a team can provide great motivation and keep you busy and active; just remember that your new exercise program involves at least half an hour, preferably every day. Don't rely on the occasional basketball game or your weekend hockey tournament.

Once you get started with regular exercise, you will be hooked. You will ask yourself why you waited so long to get into regular activity. Not only will you feel better—more alive and more alert—but exercising on a regular basis will help you to lose fat and to keep the weight off.

Exercise Alone Is Not a Replacement for Proper Eating Habits

As you get into regular exercise, it's important to understand that while exercise has many benefits, it cannot take the place of healthy eating choices. It's a male myth that you don't need to change your diet if you exercise. Exercise is part of your overall weight loss project, and you must learn to be dedicated to your new eating habits *and* your new exercise habits. You'll quickly see the compounding benefits of increased energy, increased strength, increased mental focus, lower body weight, and higher self-esteem.

Do's and Don'ts of Fitness

Starting a fitness routine should not be a chore. The following do's and don'ts will increase the effectiveness of your workout and reduce your chances of suffering from stiffness and soreness:

Do's:

- Set realistic goals and objectives. Assess your current fitness level before starting. It will help you to be realistic.
- Warm up and cool down properly—always. Stretching before and after will prevent injury and stiffness. It's worth the few extra minutes.
- Vary your routine to avoid boredom and reduce risk of injury due to overuse of a single muscle group.
- Keep a progress chart. Use the activity tracker every day. This way you'll be aware of any changes when you improve. It will be proof of your success.
- Drink plenty of water before, during, and after your workout; if you wait until you're thirsty, you've waited too long. To get the maximum benefit from your workout, you should not be dehydrated.
- Keep it convenient. Choose something that you can do almost anytime or anywhere, even if you're alone. It may be that you buy

some fitness equipment that you can use at home so you can work out while you watch TV. If you're going to join a gym or health club, choose a location that is close to either your home or your office.

· Enlist a friend. There will be days when you just won't feel like exercising; having a buddy to help motivate you is a great way to keep you going. It is best to work out with a friend who has the same interests and a similar level of fitness.

· Have the right clothing: Wearing comfortable sports shoes with good support can significantly reduce your risk of injury. Non-restrictive, breathable clothing is best for activity. Also, be sure to use safe, reliable equipment.

Don'ts:

· Don't overdo it. Injury is the main reason people quit exercising, and the most common cause of injuries is exercising too hard, or trying to do too much too soon. Whatever activity you choose, begin at a very moderate intensity and then adjust it as time goes by, according to your fitness and comfort level.

· Don't compare yourself to others or feel that you have to keep up with them. Remember that you're doing this for you and no one else.

· Don't increase duration or intensity in large amounts in any given week.

· Don't increase intensity and duration at the same time. First increase duration, then increase intensity.

· Don't overdo it in hot or humid weather.

· Don't forget to reward yourself. Buy a new pair of track shoes or a new TV for the workout room.

How to Plan Your Fitness

Here are guidelines on the intensity level of various activities:

You want to aim for moderate intensity at first, and work your way up to vigorous activity. "Moderate intensity" means activity that causes a slight but noticeable increase in breathing and heart rate. One way to gauge moderate activity is with the "talk test": exercising hard enough to break a sweat but not so hard you can't comfortably carry on a conversation.

Moderate activity	Vigorous activity	Intense activity
Walking a mile in 15–20 min (3–4 mph)	Walking briskly (5 mph) or jogging (12 min/mile)	Running/sprinting
Hiking	In-line skating	Mountain climbing
Cycling (10 mph)	Mountain biking or cycling (12 mph)	Step aerobics (6-to 8-in steps)
Yard work/gardening/ washing car by hand	Mowing lawn with hand mower/digging/ chopping wood	Circuit weight training
Swimming (slowly)	Swimming laps	Water jogging
Yoga	Low-impact aerobics	High-impact aerobics
Ballroom or square dancing	Playing squash, tennis, basketball, soccer, skiing	Jumping rope
Golfing (no cart), fishing (standing/casting)	Canoeing (briskly)	
Vacuuming	Moving furniture	
Playing actively with children		

Conquer Your Fitness Procrastination

These are some of the favorite excuses for why people can't exercise— and they are all hogwash!

No Time   This is the oldest excuse in the world. Of course you have time, because you can split the activity up throughout the day. Whether it's walking from the car (from the farthest place in the parking lot) or taking the stairs instead of the elevator, this counts as activity. When you're home you can hop on a stationary bike or the treadmill while you're watching TV. Regular exercise is one of the best stress relievers around, so give up half an hour of TV time. The key is to make exercise part of your daily plan. Set the alarm 30 minutes earlier, have a workout at lunch time, walk to and from work…just do it!

Too Tired   This is probably the worst excuse of all. Exercising will increase your energy level, and your sleeping will improve too. Constant fatigue can be a direct result of inactivity and poor nutrition.

Bad Back or Sore Knees   Chronic back pain or stiff knees can really cramp your physical activity. However, getting in shape can minimize and even eliminate back and joint pain. Weight-bearing exercise increases bone density as well as muscle mass while decreasing excess pounds. Every additional pound puts more force on your body's joints. As you lose weight and exercise, your joints will be under less stress and will become stronger.

THE IMPORTANCE OF ACTIVITY LONG-TERM

Plan carefully, and you can slowly ease yourself back into a routine and find something you enjoy. Do this as safely as possible so you do not injure yourself (which would, at best, set you back, or, at worst, put you off completely).

Just as I'm asking you to make a permanent change to your eating habits, so too am I asking you to make a permanent change to your activity level. Physical fitness cannot be stored; when you have begun an exercise program, you need to stick with it to keep the benefits. Once you start, you'll get hooked, and you'll ask yourself why you waited so long to get going.

AVOIDING SABOTAGE: STRATEGIES FOR SUCCESS

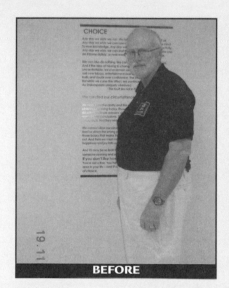

BEFORE

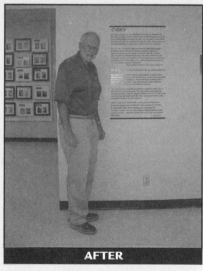

AFTER

I am a 60-year-old man and lost 50 pounds between November 2006 and June 2007; I have been stable since. In fact, my weight has been within a three-pound range from June to now. I have always fought my weight since I was 12 years old and have lost large amounts of weight five or six times in the past—each time putting it back on, and then some. I can remember driving and listening to Harvey's CDs, where he said that when we lose our weight we are still fat men but in a slim body. What we did to lose the weight is what we need to keep doing. The program is the maintenance, and this is my new mindset. The way I lost the weight is the way I need to keep eating forever. It is simple but I never got it till then. Now I know that I can maintain my weight loss by doing what I am doing every day.

Gerry Ross (a fat man in a slim body)

Changing your lifestyle on a permanent basis is a long-term project. Think of it as a marathon rather than a sprint. You're now equipped with a program; you know how to make it work. And I know that you're motivated to achieve your goals. Yet in our day-to-day lives, we need to be alert. The road to a sane eating program has ongoing risks, and they can pop up at any time.

Consider this analogy: when we're driving, we've learned to watch for pedestrians, unskilled drivers, merging traffic, slippery roads, and numerous other dangers and distractions. When we first learn to drive, it can be a hairy experience. Once we've put in the hours, and we're alert and careful about planning our route, we can feel confident of getting to our destination safely.

The difference between driving and the diet sabotage I'm going to talk about is that most things that happen on the road are beyond your control. They would have happened to anyone in that place at that time. With diet sabotage, however, you face challenges that are targeted at you specifically. Those hurdles can be set up by those who love you or work with you; sometimes by your friends; sometimes by that bad character, "Slick," who exists in each one of us.

If you have a clear understanding of the obstacles you will face, you can plan your reaction, your defensive gesture, and the firmness of your response well in advance. This will reduce the chances that you will be caught off guard, and ensure you stick with your project all the time. You're less likely to compromise.

WHAT'S WRONG WITH COMPROMISE?

If you've gained a significant amount of weight during your life, then I know for certain that you've developed some deeply ingrained unhealthy eating behaviors that are going to be hard to change. Until you've really established your new habits and had success with your project, you can't afford to compromise if you want to succeed.

The National Weight Control Registry in the United States was founded in 1994. It has between 6,000 and 6,500 registered members, who have all lost a minimum of 30 pounds and maintained it for two years. That's why it's called a weight *control* registry. They're not talking about dieters, because as we all know, dieting doesn't work. So their belief is that if people have maintained their weight for over two years, then they have actually changed their eating behavior. That is how long I'm asking you to remain totally dedicated to this project and to your new life, before you begin to allow a little more flexibility and occasional compromise. (It's true that you may slip during the two years, and if you do, you must immediately get back on your program.)

I've seen far too many men slide out of good eating habits because they didn't make it a project to succeed, and they felt it was okay to "compromise." First they make one exception, and then they make another. Soon the weight management program becomes the exception, and they have failed.

Follow the program the way that I have laid it out. As you can see from the pictures and testimonials, this way works. Don't compromise the integrity of the eating plans, because you simply can't fool around with what you are eating.

Sabotage from Those Who Are Close to You

Sabotage will come first from those people who are close to you—your family and friends. They can feel threatened, even insulted, because someone close to them is making a dramatic change. That is when they can become subversive.

Sabotage from Your Co-Dependent Eating Partner

Have you ever heard any of these phrases in your house? "Just relax—it's no fun when you focus on eating." Or "We don't have to suffer as well." Or even "How many times have you done this before? It never works!" These sentences reflect the negative thoughts of those who are not ready to help you change your life for the better, and they want to keep you just as you are, because it's comfortable and easier. Remember, change is very frightening for some people, and they will resist it.

All of us have heard of co-dependency, usually in the context of people who "support" each other in their drinking. Changing your eating choices affects a lot of people in your circle, particularly the one who is closest to you. See if these sound familiar: "Aren't you going to join me in this one piece of pie that I made just for you?" "You're not going to have a piece of your own birthday cake?" Eating together forms a bond, and you've got to replace that vehicle with other things that you can do together.

My wife, Helen, and I were co-dependent eaters. We took delight in going to fast food restaurants together, and our early marriage was warmed by endless shared plates of heavy cooking. When I had my epiphany, and committed myself to a life of healthy eating, Helen was not amused; in fact, she was insulted. I was taking a pastime that we had shared happily together and thrown it out the window.

She's not the only person to have experienced this as rejection. One day, I received a phone call from the wife of a dentist client who had lost over 80 pounds. His wife left a very heated voice mail saying that I was ruining her home and their family life because her husband was becoming "aggressive" about the way he ate! Interestingly, her husband had told me that she was grossly overweight.

I had another client whose wife threatened to leave him because he was on the program. He was changing and becoming a very good-looking man. His whole demeanor had turned around, and she was threatened. Instead of getting onboard and finding health with him, she wanted to find someone new who could keep with the same unhealthy patterns!

The saddest story ever was a 48-year-old client, a businessman called Jack. He had been sent to me by his doctor. He had high blood pressure and sleep apnea, which left him so tired during the day that he had once fallen asleep at a red light. At night he used a CPAP machine for sleep apnea. He also had back problems and was on all kinds of medications that could only be reduced if he got to the correct weight.

I provided him with all the details of my program, and suggested to him that he could benefit from one-on-one counseling sessions to help keep him on track. He told me that those would not be necessary as his wife would do it. I had learned during our initial interview that his wife was 60 pounds overweight. I looked at him in amazement. "Drinkers can't help drinkers to quit drinking," I said. I couldn't believe my ears. This man would not go to a terrible golfer to learn how to improve his swing. He was adamant with me: she would be his coach!

After seven weeks, he had lost only seven pounds. Within six weeks he had stopped attending my weekly group sessions saying to me that the program was not working for him. He admitted to me that his wife was not very supportive of all the changes; she found them too tough. Not long after, I was talking with a friend of his, and asked how he was doing. I learned to my great sadness and disappointment that within a couple of months he had died of a massive heart attack. So unnecessary, and yet not so uncommon.

Part of your project is to break free of negative, co-dependent eating habits. Make it a major focus of the program, especially in the beginning. Let your determination spill over. Don't take no for an answer. Cook enough of your healthy meals for two, and make it easy for the other person to get started. Share this book, and talk about your goals. Do whatever it takes to keep moving in the right direction yourself and to help your loved ones feel good about the changes you are making.

I was lucky because it wasn't long before my wife was just as motivated as I was, and we began to give each other real support—support in being healthy and living a long and happy life together. It didn't happen for us overnight, but we did get there. And then our commitment was unbreakable, and our shared success felt even better than succeeding alone would have. If you have a partner in eating, finding a way to break your unhealthy habits may take time and patience, but once you do, you'll have a partner in health.

Sabotage from Extended Family, Friends, and Co-Workers

Though you may not eat with these people daily, when you do, they are very likely to offer you foods you don't want any more, and to make assumptions about how you will eat based on the past. Your changes aren't happening in a vacuum: everyone around you is going to need some coaching to get used to the new you.

Tell people that you have changed. You must have a totally confident attitude or this will not work. There is no middle ground. You and your eating styles are changing forever.

Sabotage from family, friends, and co-workers can be conscious or unconscious.

I had a client named Jason. He lost 73 pounds in the first eight months of my program. He went to his parents' home filled with pride about how great he looked. They ordered Chinese food, and to his credit, he said that he was going to grab a healthy sandwich instead. He told me that rather than being proud about how well he was doing, they were very upset that he wasn't appreciative of the meal that they'd ordered for him.

Maybe you have drinking buddies and a long-standing arrangement for a night out with the guys. You feel pressured and don't want to be perceived as a wuss. Or maybe your office mates like to stop by for a chat with a few donuts. How can you, as a man who wants to become healthy, recognize and know how to face these very serious challenges to your successful completion of this project?

You've got to tell all of these people, "I just don't eat that way anymore." Tell them that you understand their love or friendship and it's important to you. Ask for their support to back you in the necessary change. That is the best way they can show their caring and friendship.

Some people will treat you as if you are already at a healthy weight after you lose just a few pounds. This is not a compliment, it is sabotage. These people will say, "What harm can a Caesar salad do? You won't fall off the wagon!" Or another favorite line: "When are you going to get back to eating normally again?" Tell them, "I'll never stop. When my body finds my level, when all my health issues are gone, and all my pills are gone, I'll still be a chronic restrained eater, and I'll never go back to my old ways."

Not everyone is going to resist your changes. In fact, some of your friends and family are going to become your best supports. Know that *you alone can do this, but you can't do this alone.* Plug into those relationships that make you feel good and offer you real support. Remember, you need those people who charge you up and give you energy. As you continue to get healthier, you'll find more and more healthy people in your world and part of your lifestyle.

Sabotage from Your Environment

I've talked about this in other chapters, but I need to say this again, because it's important: keep your home free from temptation. This doesn't mean an empty refrigerator or pantry; it means filling those places with healthy foods—fruits, non-fat yoghurts, and cut-up salads that you can use to cook nutritious meals and snacks—according to plans you've set for yourself.

Sabotage in Your Own Mind

While they're all related, the worst sabotage comes from within—from you. As you know, I call that bad guy within you "Slick."

You may have tried dieting before and failed, and maybe that's left you feeling nervous about failure. But we already know that diets don't work. Recognize that when you're changing your eating behavior, you're going to have slow weeks. There will be times when you have slower-than-average overall losses, compared to previous weeks. Don't let these times cause fear or doubt, because you're in it for the long haul. There are days when you may be a plodder, and there will be days when you feel like an all-star. Don't let Slick get the better of you by causing you to think that you're back on one of your old diets.

Even though you should now have a clear understanding on why you weren't successful, doubts may creep into the back of your mind, and those doubts can become the seeds of failure. So confront them head-on:

Fear Fear makes men disempowered. It cripples their initiative. It's like having flat tires when everything else in the car is working perfectly. In the big leagues, if a hitter is filled with fear and goes out to face a pitcher who is confident, you know who's going to win the battle. Now, it's natural for everyone to feel a certain amount of anxiety before a big event, but you can't allow it to turn into fear. Not surprisingly, the way you prevent this is by thoroughly analyzing the situation ahead of time.

Fear of Change There's the old story about water torture where a man has water dripped on his head. Initially, it drives him crazy, but if he can last long enough, he gets used to it, and if it stops he'll actually miss it. It's a sad thing, but this can happen with excess pounds. The chances are that you've become used to being overweight. You've learned to live with a fat mindset. There's no question that avoiding change keeps us comfortable. Think about a big change that you've made in your life. You've moved homes; you've got a new job or started a new business. Even though these are efforts to improve ourselves in the long run, during the period of adjustment, it's always somewhat uncomfortable. Understand that that's life. That's normal.

Use the fear of what could happen as a catalyst for change. Use that energy to propel yourself forward and to strengthen your resolve. Never again will your unhealthy lifestyle cause you fear, because you are changing. Anticipate what that change will mean to you and how it will feel. Now that you can see the future, what is there to fear about it?

Fear of Failure Success or failure is really an attitude about the things that you're doing. This may sound ridiculous, but people who are successful never really believe that they have failed, even if others do. Are they nuts, or are they on to something? What other people call failure, they merely call setbacks.

You won't fail if you don't believe that you have failed! You may have setbacks on your journey, but if you view this process as a lifelong journey, you can't fail. You may take the odd detour; perhaps you'll find that it takes you longer to get to your destination. But, with the right attitude, you'll automatically get back on track.

Aristotle said it best: "You are what you repeatedly do. Excellence is not an event—it is a habit."

Fear of Hunger If you think pizza is "to die for," keep eating the way you are now, and you will!

Look, you may say that you love steaks, but I believe that you don't love food. Food is the sustenance that allows you to focus on what you really love: your hobbies, your friends, your children, and your family.

The fact is, if you follow the program closely, you'll probably find that you're eating more regularly and having more food than you did in the past. I can tell you confidently that your fear of hunger is unjustified. And you will be learning the joy of eating foods that you have not tried before. When you start to appreciate the real taste of food, you're going to look at stuff you used to love, pizza or french fries, and wonder how you ever ate them. I have a friend who is on this program who tried something he used to love: a potato chip with high-fat, high-salt Dijon dip. He was repulsed at how greasy and disgusting it tasted. He went back to his raw vegetables with a light dip and was more satisfied than he would have ever believed. I promise you, this program would never be successful if it ever let you become hungry.

SETBACKS

First, remember that a setback is not a failure! It could be a sign that you don't have a workable plan in place. Motivation is sustained by your successes, not your slip-ups. Acknowledge that you can start over again the very same day, even at the very next meal.

Setbacks occur to everyone with everything that they are trying to accomplish. The difference between those who achieve their goals and those who don't is their attitude to those setbacks. Will you use setbacks as a reason for no longer carrying on with your program, or can you view them as lessons that will help you reach your goal? Mistakes can be the best teachers, especially in the beginning when you are learning which parts of the program are the toughest for you.

If you know baseball, then you'll understand that a great hitting average is .333. When you think about it, this means that the hitter misses two out of every three times that he goes to bat. However, every time he misses a curve ball, a fastball, or a slider, he tries to understand how he was fooled by the pitcher's arm motion in order to prevent a miss the next time. It's a process in his journey.

Let's say you missed lunch. Your kids order pizza, and you eat it. Next thing you know, you're filled with negative, chastising thoughts. You're thinking, "I give up. I can't do this." Remember that you are embarking on a lifetime weight management effort. The setbacks you encounter should not stop this effort, but focus it so that the same setbacks do not slow your progress by happening over and over again.

Harvey's Quick Rules for Overcoming Setbacks

1. Think about what happened. Did you skip breakfast or lunch? Did you eat during the day?
2. Learn from mistakes: sweeping setbacks under the rug does not help.
3. Forgive yourself quickly…*success is failure turned upside down.*
4. Get rid of or fix whatever it was that set you back.
5. Record what you ate, and where and when you ate it.
6. Put it behind you by getting right back on the program for the next meal.
7. Eat next as if nothing had happened.
8. Remember, no one can be perfect, so you haven't failed!

Plateaus

As you know, I recommend that you weigh yourself once a week, on the same scale at the same time of day. Adherence to my program and the Daily Awareness Eating Record will help you see where binges or slip-ups occur, and why. Use a highlighter each week in your record to indicate any areas that need work. Often plateaus are self-induced; we're not perfect. If you make an error or compromise, you may have neutralized any weight loss that you could have had that week. That's life; just get back on the program.

Plateaus can also be caused by what you eat the night before you weigh yourself. If you had a heavy meal or ate too late, food may still be in your body. Too much salt in your last food can also drive your weight up. This is because sodium can contain many times its weight in fluids or water.

I want to emphasize that if gains show up, don't get too hung up. This is just a small blip on the screen. There are plateaus that have no rhyme or reason. You can do everything right and still have temporary setbacks. They could be due to not having had a bowel movement, or to building muscle (which weighs more than fat).

Plateaus or temporary gains don't define you or your efforts. You're a man on a mission, and the idea is to stay on course and get yourself fit and healthy.

Apathy

Apathy usually occurs when you're depleted of energy. It results in an erosion of self-confidence. You feel as if you just don't care anymore, and ask yourself whether it's all worth the effort. A good trick here is to make yourself remember how you felt when you first started the program. Pull those envelopes out of the drawer, and re-read how you used to eat, feel, and think about the future before you started the plan. Clearly, there were some very strong motivations to change your life around. Have they gone away? Of course they haven't. Next, remind yourself that you've already successfully taken a number of steps. In effect, you're well underway. Ask yourself, "Why would I stop now?"

Often apathy sets in from too much concentration on the final result, which may remain a couple of years away. Instead, concentrate on hitting your benchmarks. For example, what simple step can you take to change your breakfast routine so that you will never again skip breakfast? Make a couple of steps in the right direction, and when you've completed them, give yourself a pat on the back. This will begin to re-establish your self-confidence. With that coming back, you'll find your energy renewed, and you can set some more small steps towards the end goal.

Celebration Sabotage

Most people feel it's time to celebrate when they lose weight. That's because they feel they've reached their goal. You must understand that you've only reached your goal when you die at your fighting weight. Celebrate every success, but learn new ways to celebrate that don't involve indulging the old habits!

Your Thoughts and Your Body

There's a great expression which I believe to be true: *If you want to know what your thoughts were like yesterday, look at your body today. If you want to know what your body will be like tomorrow, listen to your thoughts today.*

You must have a realistic understanding of how you're going to live the rest of your life. Remember that the route you choose must be attainable, maintainable, and sustainable. Understand that it's going to take two to five years to learn how to maintain and stabilize your weight at the right level. It's always going to be a learning process, and so you must value who you are, all the way through this process with its ups and downs. You must build positive thoughts today, and every day draw yourself closer to your goal.

What are your thoughts today?

CONCLUSION:
A NEW MAN FOR LIFE

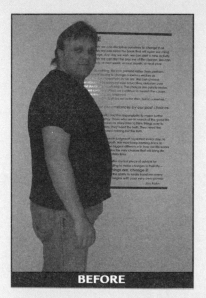

BEFORE

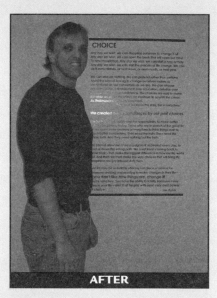

AFTER

For the better part of my life I have had issues with my weight and, more recently, concerns about my overall health and well-being. I would say the weight gain began for me quite gradually in my early twenties and progressively became worse as the years passed by. How I ever reached this point of denial and self-abuse in my life was totally beyond me.

I was quite active and physically fit in my youth, so I always felt that I could conquer extra weight by either burning it off through some rigorous exercise program or trying some newly discovered fad diet.

155

Eventually, I would avoid annual physicals with my family doctor, simply because I did not want to face the fact that I had serious health issues. Although I realized that my blood pressure was high and my cholesterol levels were not normal, I simply did not want to hear it; even worse, I wasn't doing anything about it. The amazing thing to me is how it just seemed to accumulate over time and before I knew it, I was flirting with 300 pounds. Now I had reached a new low in my life. I was depressed and thoroughly disgusted with myself; I had hit rock-bottom!

It was late December 2006 and we were coming home after having one of those gargantuan Christmas dinners that only Mom knows how to prepare. I had totally stuffed my face with food and was feeling just terrible. My wife, Anne, had noticed that I was in a real funk over this. So on January 7, 2007, I went to see Harvey and I meant business. . . I was bound and determined; failure was not an option. As I began the program I was pleasantly surprised at its simplicity and effectiveness. I found Harvey's lectures to not only be inspirational and energizing but also educational and informative. Before I knew it, the pounds started melting away; it had an enormously positive effect on my life. In about six months, I had reached my goal weight and felt amazing. I started to exercise every day and all those ailments that were bothering me just a few short months earlier were all withering away. Gone were the back pain, sore knees, and heel spurs. My doctor was also amazed at my turnaround. My blood pressure and cholesterol levels were back to normal; my heart rate had even come down, since it wasn't working as hard just to keep me alive.

I simply cannot express in a few short words the appreciation and respect I have for Harvey and this program. As a result of this experience, it is my sincere belief that maintaining my health is the most important aspect of my life. My weight loss has had a domino effect on everything—my relationships, my work, my attitude, my emotional well-being—it has all just seemed to fall into place!

Harvey, thank you for doing what you do best and giving me a new lease on life. I've lost over 80 pounds and life is good.

Aldo Galeazza

You or someone you love may have bought this book thinking that it was a diet book with a different slant because it was focused on the issue from a man's perspective. Now that you're arriving at the last chapter, you have realized that it's not a diet book at all.

It's a book about how eating has had a dramatic effect on the person you are. It's a book that's suggesting that your eating has probably caused you to be a lesser individual than you might have been at this point in your life if only you had managed it better. It's a book that's challenging you to become a "chronic restrained eater." It's a book that says you can choose to eat well, buying foods that are available at the grocery store, and that you never need to feel hungry to be healthy for the rest of what should be a much longer life. It's a book about discovering the truly great man that you are meant to be.

If you're reading this book, then it's my suspicion that you have allowed eating to change who you are in a negative way. Is there a part of you that still doesn't want to admit that there's a problem? A part of you that thinks I'm wrong? Maybe you still think that things are okay and that you're doing just fine, thank you. I think that's crap. It's true that I don't know you, but in my 30-plus years of counseling overweight men, I've discovered that none are truly happy inside. There isn't one of them that doesn't ultimately admit that he wishes he looked and felt like he did when he was at his peak as a younger person. I've also seen that when they change their lives and find their appropriate weight again, they really do become reinvigorated, and start acting like that previously faraway and forgotten person.

Why is this important to me? Because I believe in the innate potential in men. I think that we can accomplish all kinds of things if we can perform at our peak. I know how my life changed when I got control of my eating, and I know from personal experience how it can destroy a man to lose control.

On the surface, excess weight distorts how you look. When this happens, I know that it affects how others view you and react to you. I ask the men I counsel, "What do you think of other men who are overweight?"

The answer always comes back the same: "They're out of control." They say it in different ways, but they're unanimous in the belief that if you can't control your weight, then you can't control your life!

I believe that when you're overweight, you may not admit it, but deep down you have a visceral understanding of this fact and that it affects whether you're truly happy about who you are. This has got to affect your self-esteem. In the end, you cannot be the truly great person that you could be for yourself, your family, your friends, and your business associates.

How you look is of course just an exterior snapshot of what's happening inside your body. Your gray skin tone, the bags under your eyes, and your signs of fatigue are all indications of what is going on inside. Ask a surgeon about what they see when they open a fat person for a routine operation. Of course, you don't need to, because if you really think about it, you already know the answer. It's not a pretty thought, and we don't tend to pay much attention to our insides, unless we're in pain or can't function normally. We always think that it's going to be the other guy! Maybe you're not ill yet, but you know it's just a matter of time. All those muscles and organs are what support us, day in and day out. What we put in our mouths each day determines whether that incredible machine, the body, works efficiently or not.

We know that if we poured impure gasoline or oil in our car, it would quickly break down. How is it that we can apply rational thought to the care of our car and not to the care of our body? When you feel bloated and overweight, when your belt is straining, when you're short of breath going upstairs or from the car to the office, your body is signaling that it is in distress!

So maybe you're still saying to yourself, "I can live with all of that, because it's my mind that counts. It's that magical soul of mine that is carrying on regardless of the body that carries it." I don't buy it, and neither should you. Your brain is a physical part of your body, and if you're healthy and fit, you're going to be able to think more clearly. What about that magical soul of yours? If you're running on high-octane fuel, you'll be able to idle at a very low rate without stalling. You'll be able to meditate or pray (whatever you want to do or call it) without the distraction of your overweight body preventing your relaxation.

Look at yourself in the mirror and decide whether you really like what you see. Then I want you to find it within yourself to eat differently for the rest of your life.

Whether you're grossly overweight, or simply need to lose the 10 or 15 pounds that have been creeping to a gradually larger number over the last few years, the chances are good that you've been quite willing to accept yourself as an overweight man with a fat mindset.

Oh, you've made half-hearted attempts to get your weight under control. You may have gone on an all-protein diet for a while. What man doesn't like protein? But you don't really expect it to work, because. . . well, there were lots of reasons!

Your parents used to make you finish everything on your plate, and while that habit didn't seem to hurt when you were young, it is hurting now. Maybe they got you hooked on treats like ice cream, cake, and cookies. That's how you were rewarded for being good, and you learned to reward yourself in the same way. Now when you're having a tough day at work, you take a break and get yourself a chocolate bar.

Maybe it's just genetic! Your dad's a big guy and you're becoming just like him in your later years, and he's mostly had a good life, hasn't he? But maybe he hasn't. Maybe he battled or is battling diseases that he wouldn't have faced if he'd been able to stay at his fighting weight all of his life.

Maybe you want to blame it on your family: all those readily available and wonderful lasagnas with a supporting cast of Caesar salad and garlic bread.

Maybe the problem is that you don't have to strain a muscle to make money any more. You're caught sitting at a desk or behind a piece of machinery and you don't have time with your job and family responsibilities to exercise more than once a month.

Maybe it's a case of not being able to escape from your ethnic heritage. Maybe you're Greek, and eating is a big part of your life. But I'm Jewish, and we love our desserts—and the Germans love their sausages; and Italians eat pasta. It doesn't matter what your background is; the chances are that food is a big part of your celebrations and culture, because way back when it was scarce, it was natural to celebrate with lots of food.

But in our society today, food is not scarce. We can have a feast at every meal for every day of the week.

So, really, it's society's fault, right? There's so much food available and it's now so fattening, how can a guy avoid it? You're caught traveling for business; entertaining is part of how you make your living. Wings and fries are one of the few rewards when you get away with the guys during the week. When you take your kids for a Big Mac, of course you're going to bond with them by having one yourself. After all, what man has time to cook, and to read the labels on food when picking up prepared food at the supermarket?

Or perhaps it's my favorite excuse: stress! Life is so stressful today, and the only way you can cope with stress is by eating. But didn't our relatives go through a war and Depression? Did they not regularly face the destruction of their crops by drought or pests? Were they not faced with incurable diseases like polio and smallpox attacking their kids, at a time when there was limited medical care and no insurance?

Stress is an inevitable part of our human existence, and we have to learn to stop complaining and discover how to be self-reliant.

Of course we have stress, but do you really think that it can be relieved by food? Stress can never be relieved by food or drink or drugs or other damaging substances. Eating poorly and excessively is substance abuse. Just because it doesn't get the negative publicity of smoking or being an alcoholic, it's equally self-destructive if you're eating too much. Further, eating the wrong kinds of food will actually increase stress. The way to work through your stress in life is with exercise, rest, meditation, and by talking it through with someone you trust.

It's time for you to take responsibility for dealing with your daily challenges. No one likes complainers. Worse yet are those who don't complain, who say they are coping and shouldering all the problems themselves, when really they're eating or drinking themselves into the hospital. I've heard all the excuses that men use for allowing themselves to become fat and soft. I know that it's BS and deep down so do you! It's time to come clean with yourself. It's time you start to use your yesterdays as teachers. Your past is only valuable if you learn to accept your mistakes, and eliminate your weaknesses.

When we allow ourselves to become overweight, our bodies are in a state of disease. If you continue to gain weight, you'll never know the day you might have lived to if you had only looked after yourself.

The way you look today is a result of the thoughts you had yesterday. If you want to know what your body will be like tomorrow, then you've got to pay attention to your thoughts today. Ask yourself, "Am I going to continue to put up with this?" "What am I going to do about this?" The answer has to be "make a change in your eating habits," starting this moment.

I truly believe that tomorrow is ours to live as we choose, and choose we must. You need your health to continue giving to your world. Don't cop out by thinking how you've got great life insurance and your family will be well looked after. They're not looked after if you're not there to provide wisdom, support, and companionship. You're not a shoulder of support for your friends if you're not around when they have problems. You can't help your favorite charities if you're not there to volunteer your time.

You've got to start looking out for number one, and that number one is you. You cannot be any use to others, if you're not in good shape yourself. Self-nourishment is the best place to focus.

Our lives are full of blessings. Any blame for things not being as they should stops with you. It's way past the time when you need to put yourself in charge of your own destiny and become your own number one fan. When you start looking out for number one, you are no longer a physical or mental burden on anyone else. You no longer have to rely on doctors because you can become your own personal health care provider.

Don't worry about it being selfish! It brings benefits to everyone. It secures their lives for as long as you're around, and by changing your eating habits, you're dramatically increasing the odds that you're going to be around for a long, long time. After all, it's the healthy stallion that can lead the herd. It's the well-fueled and maintained engine that can pull the other cars on the train.

Of course the first week will be tough, but you can learn to reward yourself with things other than food. When you've stayed away from fried foods, white flour, white sugar, and excess fats for a while, you won't even miss them. In fact, you'll wonder what ever attracted you to them in the first place. Not only is it exhilarating to get rid of the toxins in your food, but you'll find it uplifting to get rid of the toxic people.

You see, I believe that there are two kinds of people: batteries included, and batteries not included. The batteries included people are full of energy, and help you to achieve the things that are important for you in your life. Then there are the batteries not included. They want to plug into you and drag you down. They don't want you to change because your ability to improve yourself would leave them with no excuse as to why they have not tried to improve their lives. If you fail, it justifies their lack of resolve. Please distance yourself from them, and surround yourself with those that are full of positive energy. You will feed off of it and you will love it.

Replace your eating habits with new things that you've never tried before. Ride a bike, paint, walk, learn a new instrument. Volunteer somewhere where they can benefit from your efforts. Life will be truly rewarding for you and you will begin to love it the way you did when you were experiencing it as a child, with boundless energy and curiosity.

You can create your own self-fulfilling prophesy. We are the result of our own minds and efforts; if we want to change, all we need to do is develop new behaviors into our daily routine.

You've now got the secrets to protecting your existence. Show respect for yourself. Your unique DNA makes you a unique human being.

Please, please use the program outlined in this book to make yourself the man that you were meant to be—a proud and fit leader for your family and community.

I SEE MYSELF

I see myself as no one can,
with all my faults and strengths as a man.

I'm a dad, a brother, a husband, son, and friend,
I'll be a picture of health 'til my long life's end.

I've climbed mountains in life and conquered many peaks,
but there is lots left to do in goals that I seek.

I look to my Future, wondering what years it will span
I'm more confident now that I've focused on a plan.

In the past there was uncertainty, discomfort, and despair
I just did not think a healthy life would be there.

My health and my future were foggy and at risk,
but now I know if only I persist,

I am able to control my greatest wealth:
the ability to dictate my personal health.

Good-bye to the pills, the threats of early demise,
I'm growing in knowledge as I'm shrinking in size.

I'm on course, I'm focused, I've got a new will,
because with each passing day, I've got more healthy skills.

My future looks brighter because I've taken command
of the most important possession I have as a man.

My body grows healthier, because I know I'm in control—
Why Not? It's my life-support system for my soul.

So as the months slip away off the calendar of time
I know in myself that a healthy life will be mine.

I see myself.

—*Harvey Brooker, December 11, 2005*

PART 3

ONE80 PLAN RECIPES FOR WEIGHT LOSS AND LIFE SUCCESS

BREAKFAST RECIPES

SCRAMBLED EGGS WITH HERBS
2 Grain Units, 2 Protein Units, 1 Free Unit, and 1 Milk Unit

- 2 slices whole wheat bread, toasted
- 2 omega-3 eggs, scrambled
- ½ tsp. dried basil or 2 tbsp. chopped fresh basil
- ½ tsp. dried oregano
- 1 tsp. sugar-free jam
- 1 cup skim milk (less 2 tbsp. for the scrambled eggs)

Preparation

In a small bowl, beat together 2 eggs and 2 tablespoons skim milk. In microwave, cook on high, stirring once or twice, about 1 to 1½ minutes. Stir. If necessary, cover with plastic wrap and let stand until eggs are fully cooked, about 1 minute.

FRENCH TOAST
2 Grain Units, 2 Protein Units, 2 Free Units, and ¼ Milk Unit

- 2 slices whole grain bread
- 1 omega-3 egg
- 2 slices turkey bacon
- 2 oz. skim milk
- 2 tsp. sugar-free syrup
- Worcestershire sauce

Preparation

Beat the egg with milk and Worcestershire. Soak one side of bread in egg mixture and then turn bread carefully to soak other side. Lightly coat non-stick skillet or grill with cooking spray. Cook egg-soaked bread on medium heat until the bread is golden brown on each side. Serve with maple syrup.

EGGS'N MUFFIN
2 Grain Units, 2 Protein Units, 1 Fruit Unit, and 1 Milk Unit

- 2 slices whole wheat English muffin, toasted
- 2 poached omega-3 eggs
- ¾ cup low-fat plain yoghurt
- 1 cup strawberries

Pour ⅓ cup water into a small bowl, then break and slip in two eggs. Gently prick yolks with tip of knife or wooden pick. Cover with plastic wrap. Microwave on full power for about 1½ to 2 minutes. If necessary, let stand, covered, until whites are completely set and yolks begin to thicken but are not hard, about 1 to 2 minutes. Lift out with slotted spoon and place on toasted English muffin. Mix the strawberries with the yoghurt.

VEGGIE OMELET

2 Grain Units, 2 Protein Units, Anytime Vegetable Units, and 1 Milk Unit

- · 2 slices whole wheat bread, toasted
- · 2 omega-3 eggs
- · ½ red pepper, chopped
- · ¼ cup mushrooms, sliced
- · 1 cup skim milk

Preparation

Cook the vegetables in a non-stick pan with a thin layer of vegetable spray, about 5 minutes. Beat the eggs with 2 tbsps. of milk and add to the vegetables. Cook on medium heat until eggs are fully cooked; serve with toast and milk.

RAISIN BREAD FRENCH TOAST

2 Grain Units, 2 Protein Units, 1 Free Unit, 1 Fruit Unit, and 1 Milk Unit

- · 2 slices raisin bread
- · 1 omega-3 egg
- · 1 oz. Canadian back bacon
- · ½ cup raspberries
- · 2 tsp. sugar-free syrup or jam
- · 1 cup skim milk
- · pinch of cinnamon

Preparation

Beat the egg with milk. Soak one side of bread in egg mixture and then turn bread carefully to soak the other side. Lightly coat non-stick skillet or grill with cooking spray. Cook egg-soaked bread on medium heat until bread is golden brown on each side. Serve with maple syrup. Grill the bacon and serve with the French toast, topped with raspberries and maple syrup or jam.

NEW MEXICO BREAKFAST

2 Grain Units, 2 Protein Units, and Anytime Vegetable Units

- 1 large whole wheat, high-fiber tortilla
- 1 omega-3 egg, scrambled
- ½ cup kidney beans, mashed
- ½ green or red pepper, chopped
- ¼ onion, chopped
- handful of cilantro or parsley, chopped
- dash Tabasco

Preparation

Cook the vegetables in a non-stick pan with a thin layer of vegetable spray, about 5 minutes. Beat the egg and add to the vegetables. Cook on medium heat until eggs are fully cooked. Spread beans on the tortilla shell and top with egg and vegetable mixture. Serve with a few shakes of Tabasco sauce.

BREAKFAST MEDLEY

2 Grain Units, 2 Protein Units, 1 Milk Unit and 1 Fruit Unit

- 2 oz. Special K cereal
- ½ cup low-fat cottage cheese
- 1 cup skim milk
- ½ cup chopped pineapple (canned, packed in its own juice)

Preparation

Mix the pineapple with the cottage cheese.

LUNCH RECIPES

OPEN-FACED SALMON SANDWICH
2 Grain Units and 2 Protein Units

- · 1 small can salmon, packed in water
- · 2 oz. whole wheat bread
- · sliced tomato and cucumber; leaf lettuce

Preparation

Spread salmon on whole wheat bread and top with Anytime Vegetables.

TUNA MELT TOASTIE
2 Grain Units and 2 Protein Units

- · 1 oz. tuna, seasoned
- · 1 oz. grated low-fat mozzarella cheese
- · 2 oz. toasted whole wheat baguette
- · onion and celery, chopped
- · tomato, sliced
- · dash of lemon juice
- · fresh basil, chopped
- · salt and pepper

Preparation

Preheat oven to "Broil." In a medium-sized bowl mix tuna, onion, celery, lemon, basil, salt, and pepper. Spread mixture on baguette and top with sliced tomato and cheese. Place in oven until cheese is melted, less than 5 minutes.

TURKEY ON PUMPERNICKEL
2 Grain Units and 2 Protein Units

- · 2 oz. lean, deli-sliced turkey
- · 2 oz. pumpernickel or rye bread
- · baby spinach or romaine, chopped
- · tomato, sliced

Preparation

Place meat on bread and top with Anytime Vegetables.

GRILLED CHICKEN SALAD
2 Grain Units, 2 Protein Units, and 1 Free Unit

- 2 oz. grilled chicken breast
- baby spinach and romaine, chopped
- mushrooms, sliced
- bean sprouts
- 1 tbsp. diet ranch-style dressing
- 1 small whole wheat, high-fiber roll

Preparation

Toss chicken with vegetables and ranch dressing. Spread evenly across the whole wheat roll.

WEEKENDER—BEAN SALAD MEDLEY
2 Grain Units, 2 Protein Units and 1 Fat Unit

- ½ cup canned chickpeas, rinsed and drained
- ½ cup canned red kidney beans, rinsed and drained
- Anytime Vegetables, chopped (red pepper, cucumber, carrots, Italian parsley, etc.)
- 1 tsp. red wine vinegar
- 2 tsp. extra virgin olive oil
- whole grain bagel, toasted

Preparation

Toss beans with vegetables, oil, and vinegar; serve with toasted bagel.

TENDER TURKEY & CRANBERRY SUB
2 Grain Units, 2 Protein Units, and 1 Sanity Saver

- 2 oz. deli-sliced turkey breast
- 2 oz. whole wheat submarine
- 2 tbsp. cranberry sauce
- coleslaw mix (pre-packaged)

- 2 tsp. apple cider vinegar
- ½ tsp. celery seed

Preparation

In a small bowl, add vinegar and celery seed to coleslaw; stir to combine. Place turkey and cranberry sauce on submarine bun and serve with salad.

WEEKENDER—HAWAIIAN CHUNKY CHICKEN PIZZA
2 Protein Units, 2 Grain Units, and 1 Fruit Unit

- 1½ oz. cooked chicken or ham, chopped
- ½ oz. shredded low-fat mozzarella cheese
- 2 small whole wheat pitas
- tomatoes, diced
- green pepper, chopped
- ½ cup chopped pineapple (packed in its own juice)

Preparation

Layer chicken or ham, cheese, tomato, green pepper, and pineapple on pitas; then top with cheese and warm in the microwave, about 15 seconds.

HAM & CHEESE
2 Protein Units, 2 Grain Units

- 1 oz. Black Forest ham
- 1 oz. light Swiss cheese
- 2 oz. whole wheat bun
- coleslaw mix (pre-packaged)
- 2 tsp. apple cider vinegar
- ½ tsp. celery seed

Preparation

In a small bowl, add vinegar and celery seed to coleslaw and stir. Place ham and cheese on whole wheat bun and serve with salad.

DINNER RECIPES

GRILLED SALMON WITH HERBS
5 Protein Units and 1 Starch Unit

- 5 oz. salmon fillet
- 1 clove garlic, minced
- ¼ cup chopped fresh dill or ½ tsp. dried dill
- ½ cup brown rice
- broccoli, chopped

Preparation

Preheat oven to 450 degrees. Add 1 cup water to the rice in a medium-sized pot, and bring water to a boil. Immediately turn heat to low and simmer until the water is gone, about 45 minutes. While rice is cooking, wash and chop the broccoli and set aside in a steamer. Place salmon on a cookie sheet or in any oven-proof pan and sprinkle with garlic and dill. When rice is fully cooked, remove from heat, leaving the lid on. Place the salmon in the oven and bake for 10 to 12 minutes, depending on thickness of fillet. Fish is done when it flakes easily with a fork. Broccoli will cook in 3–4 minutes over steam. Do not overcook fish or vegetables!

LIME-GLAZED CHICKEN
5 Protein Units, 1 Starch Unit, and 1 Dinner Vegetable Unit

- 5 oz. grilled chicken breast, boneless, no skin
- 1 small baked potato
- 2 tbsp. salsa
- ½ cup corn niblets
- 1 cup chicken broth
- Anytime Vegetables (chopped carrots, celery, zucchini, and/or tomatoes)
  Marinade (makes enough for 4 chicken breasts)
- 2 tbsp. olive oil
- ¼ cup Dijon mustard
- 1 tsp. dried tarragon
- juice of 1 lime, plus rind (finely grated)
- 1 clove garlic, minced

Preparation

Mix glaze ingredients. Place chicken breasts in baking dish and marinate overnight. Remove chicken from marinade; discard marinade. Preheat oven to 350 degrees. Wash the potato and prick with a fork; then put it in the oven for about 45 minutes, or until cooked. In a small saucepan, heat the chicken broth and add vegetables to make a simple soup. Bake chicken for 18–25 minutes, until fully cooked through, and serve with baked potato, salsa, corn, and soup.

TERIYAKI CHICKEN
5 Protein Units, 1 Starch Unit, 1 Fat Unit, and 1 Sanity Saver

- 5 oz. boneless, skinless chicken breast, thinly sliced
- broccoli, chopped
- red and green pepper, sliced
- onion, chopped
- mini-carrots, peeled
- 1 tsp. canola oil
- 2 tbsp. teriyaki sauce
- ½ cup brown rice

Preparation

Bring 1 cup of water to boil and add rice. Reduce heat to low and simmer until cooked—about 45 minutes. Heat oil in wok or skillet at medium heat. Sauté vegetables for 4 to 5 minutes and set aside. Brown chicken in skillet until no longer pink (5–8 minutes). Return vegetables to skillet with teriyaki sauce and toss to coat. Serve over rice.

CATALAN FISH WITH MUSHROOMS (SERVES 4)
5 Protein Units and 1 Starch Unit

- 1 lb. sole fillets
- 1 tbsp. extra virgin olive oil
- 1 lb. mini/gourmet button mushrooms or sliced button mushrooms
- 4 cloves garlic, minced
- ¼ cup Italian parsley, chopped
- ¼ tsp. each salt and pepper
- ¼ cup water
- 2 tbsp. sherry vinegar

Roasted Red Pepper Sauce:

- ½ cup roasted red peppers (in a jar)
- 1 tsp. extra virgin olive oil
- 1 tbsp. sherry vinegar

Preparation

Roasted Red Pepper Sauce: In blender or food processor, puree peppers, oil, and vinegar until smooth. Set aside.

Sole: In a large non-stick skillet, heat oil over medium-high heat and cook mushrooms, garlic, parsley, and half each of the salt and pepper for about 8 minutes, stirring occasionally or until golden brown. Add water and vinegar and bring to boil.

Place sole fillets on top of mushrooms and sprinkle with remaining salt and pepper. Cover skillet and steam for about 4 minutes or until fish flakes easily with fork. Divide fish and mushrooms onto plates and drizzle each plate with Roasted Red Pepper Sauce.

Other options: Monkfish, tuna, or swordfish can be used.

PORK TENDERLOIN WITH FENNEL
5 Protein Units, 1 Starch Unit, and 1 Fat Unit

- 5 oz. pork tenderloin
- 1 small baked potato
- 1 tsp. olive oil
- 1 garlic clove, minced
- ¼ tsp. fennel seeds
- cooked fennel or steamed cauliflower

Preparation

Rub pork with garlic clove and fennel seeds. Brush pork with olive oil. Season with salt and pepper.

- To barbecue: Grill on medium-high heat, turning frequently, about 20 minutes.
- To bake: Preheat oven to 425 degrees. Roast in oven until pork is cooked through, about 25 minutes. Let pork rest 5 minutes. Thinly slice pork crosswise.
- To cook fennel: Trim off fronds. Cut into 8 long chunks. Cook in boiling water for 8 minutes.

CHICKEN CHIMICHANGA CASSEROLE (MAKES 2 SERVINGS)

5 Protein Units

- 2 boneless, skinless chicken breasts, chopped (about 8 oz.)
- 1 tsp. vegetable oil
- 1 small red onion, finely chopped
- 1 package (8 oz.) mushrooms, sliced
- 1 jalapeno pepper, seeded and diced*
- 1 clove garlic, minced
- ¼ cup low-sodium chicken broth
- 1 tsp paprika or chilli powder
- Salt and pepper to taste
- 1 package (6 oz.) baby spinach, washed
- ½ cup shredded light cheddar cheese

*Buy sliced jalapenos in a jar

Preparation

Preheat oven to broil. In large non-stick skillet, heat oil over medium-high heat and cook onion, mushrooms, jalapeno, and garlic for about 8 minutes or until mushrooms are golden. Add chicken, broth, and paprika and cook, stirring, for 6 minutes, until chicken is fully cooked and no longer pink inside. Add salt and pepper to taste. Scrape into small shallow casserole dish.

Return skillet to medium-high heat and lightly cook spinach for about 2 minutes or until wilted. Spread spinach over top of chicken mixture, sprinkle with cheese, and broil in oven for about 3 minutes or until cheese is melted and bubbly. Serve over brown rice.

Leftovers are delicious for lunch the next day.

CHICKEN PARMIGIANA LITE

5 Protein Units and 1 Starch Unit

- 4 oz. cooked boneless, skinless chicken breast
- 1 oz. low-fat ricotta cheese or low-fat mozzarella cheese
- ½ cup cooked whole-wheat spaghetti
- ½ cup tomatoes, chopped
- dash of pepper

- ¼ tsp. oregano
- pinch of garlic powder
- steamed asparagus or green beans (make extra for breakfast leftovers)

Preparation

Preheat oven to 350 degrees. Place chicken breast in a shallow baking dish. Blend the pepper and oregano with the cheese. Rub chicken with garlic powder. Spoon cheese mixture and crushed tomatoes in center of each breast. Bake for 20–30 minutes. Serve on top of spaghetti.

HEARTY MEAT & BEAN CHILLI (MAKES 4 SERVINGS)
5 Protein Units and 1 Starch Unit

- 8 oz. extra-lean ground turkey or chicken
- 1 tsp. vegetable oil
- 1 stalk celery, chopped
- 1 large carrot, chopped
- 1 onion, chopped
- 2 cloves garlic, minced
- 1 tbsp. chilli powder
- ½ tsp. each ground cumin and dried oregano
- 1 can (28 oz) diced tomatoes or stewed chilli-style tomatoes
- 1 cup canned black beans, drained and rinsed
- 1 green pepper, chopped
- salt and pepper to taste
- 2 cups brown rice, cooked

Preparation

In saucepan, heat oil over medium heat and cook celery, carrot, onion, garlic, chilli powder, cumin, and oregano for 5 minutes or until softened. Add meat and cook, stirring, for 5 minutes or until no longer pink.

Add tomatoes, beans, and pepper and bring to a boil. Reduce heat and simmer, stirring often, for about 20 minutes or until thickened. Add salt and pepper to taste, if needed. Serve over rice.

INDEX

nutrition (key to ONE80 plan), 100

turkey recipes (*Continued*)

Tender Turkey & Cranberry Sub,
176–77

Turkey on Pumpernickel, 175

type 2 diabetes, 13, 20, 23, 37, 41

units

additional, 112, 114

allowed, 111

daily target, 111

for food types, 114–18

free, 112, 118

replacement, 112

unit values, 110–11

uric acid, 39

USDA Food Guide Pyramid, 111

vacations, 97–98

value, as a person, 64–65

variety, of foods, 85–86, 124

vegetable oils, 109

vegetable protein, 106–7

vegetables, 88, 104–5, 109

"anytime," 104–5, 112, 114, 117, 121

"dinner," 105, 114, 117, 122, 181

vigorous activity, 141

visceral fat, 38

visualization, 72–73

waist circumference, 19, 38, 127

Waitley, Denis, 67

walking, 135, 136–37

water, 85, 124, 139

WebMD, 37

weddings, 96

weekly menu, quick reference, 126

weighing your food, 84, 91, 119

weighing yourself, 83, 127–28, 153

weight, graphing, 12, 14

weight fluctuations, 83

weight gain

around abdomen, 19–20

impacts of, 13–14, 36

increasing over lifetime, 10–12

and physical appearance, 158

and sexual performance, 46–50

and stress, 160

temporary, 153

weight loss

benefits of, 101

calorie deficit needed, 101

goals, 68

previous attempts at, 159

principles, 71–77

as a project, 64–77

rate of, 102

and regular physical activity, 134

support for, 24–25

weight loss industry, 52–53

groups aimed at women, 58

weight loss products, 55–56

weight loss resorts, 57

weight training, 134, 136, 137–38

Wiener, Kevin (story), 63–64

woks, 91

women

different from men, 21, 37–38, 58

pressured to be thin, 21

work

advancing at, 34

emotions at, 29

energy to perform, 43–44

yearly review, of weight loss project, 71